D0212477

HEALTH CARE'S
FORGOTTEN MAJORITY

HEALTH CARE'S FORGOTTEN MAJORITY

Nurses and Their Frayed White Collars

Jacqueline Goodman-Draper

AUBURN HOUSE
Westport, Connecticut • London

TEXAS STATE TECH. COLLEGE
LIBRARY-SWEETWATER TX.

Library of Congress Cataloging-in-Publication Data

Goodman-Draper, Jacqueline.
    Health care's forgotten majority : nurses and their frayed white
collars / Jacqueline Goodman-Draper.
      p. cm.
    Includes bibliographical references and index.
    ISBN 0–86569–248–3
    1. Nursing—Social aspects. 2. Professional socialization.
3. Trade-unions—Nurses. 4. Class consciousness. 5. Occupational
prestige. 6. Role conflict. 7. Nurses—Psychology. 8. Hospitals—
Sociological aspects. I. Title.
RT86.5.G66   1995
610.73'06'9—dc20   95–3751

British Library Cataloguing in Publication Data is available.

Copyright © 1995 by Jacqueline Goodman-Draper

All rights reserved. No portion of this book may be
reproduced, by any process or technique, without
the express written consent of the publisher.

Library of Congress Catalog Card Number: 95–3751
ISBN: 0–86569–248–3

First published in 1995

Auburn House, 88 Post Road West, Westport, CT 06881
An imprint of Greenwood Publishing Group, Inc.

Printed in the United States of America

The paper used in this book complies with the
Permanent Paper Standard issued by the National
Information Standards Organization (Z39.48–1984).

10 9 8 7 6 5 4 3 2 1

Copyright Acknowledgments

The author and publisher gratefully acknowledge permission for use of the following material:

Susan M. Reverby, *Ordered to Care: The Dilemma of American Nursing, 1850–1945* (New York:
Cambridge University Press, 1987). Copyright © Susan M. Reverby. Reprinted with the permission
of Cambridge University Press.

Susan M. Reverby, "The Nursing Disorder: A Critical History of the Hospital-Nursing Relationship,
1860–1945." Ph.D. dissertation, Boston University, 1982. Reprinted with the permission of the author.

Contents

970109

Illustrations

Preface

After college and prior to my graduate training, I landed my first job: a clinical electromyographic technician at one of New York's most prestigious neurological institutes, giving electric shocks to patients, to test for neuromuscular disease. After the initial thrill (and fear) of my duties had worn off, this job--highly routinized and dead-ended--subjected me to a rude awakening. Despite the fact that I had just graduated from Barnard College--where we were socialized to believe that the sea would part for us the moment the school's name was mentioned--and that my father was a research scientist at this medical center, I was treated as simply a technician, stripped of my other class accoutrements: a certain status concordant with my education. Physicians would speak in our presence as though we were invisible. My boss, a physician of British descent, would not even acknowledge us in public.

The head technician of the lab in which I worked was Betty Jean Hughley, an impressive African-American woman from Alabama. She had been rejected by all the northern medical schools to which she had applied and, try as she might, was unable to obtain assistance for entrance from the physicians in our lab. She introduced me to the hospital's union, Local 1199, of which I was an automatic member but had no real interest initially. Despite the fact that I knew I would eventually leave the hospital, I felt a sense of security with that union. Hughley went on to become an organizer for the union and is currently one of its executive vice presidents. It is primarily because of my experience in the lab and my friendship with Betty Jean that I went on to study the health care labor process and its relationship to class identity and collective organization.

During the process of writing this book, I incurred many other debts, not least of which is to Katherine Newman. She tried to soften my tendency toward stilted academic prose, to focus my thoughts and sharpen my ideas. She read several drafts, editing and reediting, barely leaving a line untouched. I can only hope that

I am perceived as caring and diligent with my students as she has been with me.

Susan Reverby showed enthusiasm for my project and provided assistance early on, during the proposal writing stage. Don Palmer also extended his generous support during the early phases of this project. He meticulously read my work and offered extremely insightful suggestions, all during his feverish publishing craze at Stanford. Rick Guarasci and Bob Schwartz believed in my work and were patient enough to listen to its various phases during a course we taught together at St. Lawrence University on the history and politics of the American workplace. I thank Robb Burlage, Sumner Rosen, and Debra Ness (for her research grant and in-kind support via Service Employees International Union). I owe no small intellectual debt to Eleanor Leacock, with whom I studied Marx in a small reading group she organized at the City of New York Graduate Center.

The contributions of the nurses who took me into their homes and who spoke to me during their lunch hours and after work hours are clearly crucial. In order to protect their anonymity, I have used pseudonyms for both the nurses and the hospitals in which they work.

My husband, Alan Draper, deserves a special award for his perseverance, good humor, and extra child care duty he took on during this arduous process. His initial reading and rereading of the manuscript was invaluable to me. Our children, Sam and Rachel, have remained a total joy throughout, putting up with their mother's preoccupation with her "other baby."

This book, although he never got a chance to read it as a finished product, is dedicated to the memory of my father, Irving Goodman--and his love of ideas, pursuit of truth, and its use for real people--and to my mother, Marion Goodman, who has always been supportive of my efforts. It is dedicated as well to my brothers, Alex, Steve, and Ben, for their humor and their unflagging support of my endeavors over the years.

I thank William Merwin, president of Potsdam College, State University of New York for granting me a research leave, and I thank Jackie Rush, Sociology Department secretary, for her meticulous typing, editing and ever present good humor amidst the constant departmental clamor. Finally, I am grateful to the National Science Foundation for its generous support of this project in 1985-86.

Chapter 1

Introduction

We're a profession? That's what they tell us. What other profession do
you know that does heavy labor? We lift, we carry, we make beds. . . . It's
hard physical labor, continually running. . . . Yet they call it a profession.
  Besides taking care of patients, I'm working to put shoes on my son's
feet. . . . I work to support my life outside this hospital.

Health care is undergoing a major transformation. The United States still spends
a greater portion of its gross national product (GNP) on health care than any other
country in the world (14 percent of the gross domestic product), with 20 percent
going to administrative costs alone (Gilbert, 1990: 33). The Clinton administration has proposed its own remedy, a system of managed competition,[1] in an effort
to drive that spending back down to 9 or 10 percent of the economy while
providing universal coverage as well (Eckholm, 1993: 270). No one knows what
the future holds.

  While physicians, hospitals, and insurance companies continue to feast at the
health care banquet, there are layers of health care workers beneath this level that
have gone hungry. Nursing aides, for example, are still paid close to the minimum
wage of $4.25 an hour, and registered nurses' average annual salaries of $24,127
compared to the average annual physician salary of $170,600 (Eckholm, 1993:
75; U.S. Bureau of Labor Statistics, 1993).

  Will this medical profession's "forgotten majority"--the educated, wage-
earning "professional" white collar worker, such as registered nurse Mary Anne
Silver quoted at the start of this chapter--still remain forgotten in this health care
hoopla? Mary Anne Silver is but one of that cadre of white collar workers,
promised, yet generally denied, professional status and its concomitant social and
economic status.

  The white collar workforce in the United States has grown considerably since
the turn of the century, with the majority of workers finding employment in large,

bureaucratic organizations. It is a group that is frequently misunderstood and ignored; among its members, many are depressed and angry. It is also a group that has given rise to many debates on how to characterize this workforce.

At a time when health care issues dominate the evening news, popular journals, and newspaper headlines, it seems worthwhile to study the occupation of nursing as a representative of the growing ranks of white collar service workers. This study therefore examines the response of white collar workers to conditions of work in the hospital, the large bureaucratic maze in which they labor, by focusing on their organizational choices: do they identify with organized labor or with individualized forms of social mobility? The answer to this question enables us to understand the consciousness or subjective dimension of this group of professionals. Do they share some kind of unified "white collar" identity, vision, or ideology?

THE CASE OF THE WHITE COLLAR WORKER

The growth of the white collar workforce in the United States has soared since the turn of the century, when it comprised a mere 4 percent of the total population. By 1959 this group had reached 40 percent of all employment and by 1985 74 percent (U.S. Bureau of the Census, 1985; Newman, 1988). The increase has resulted in large part from changes in the organization of work. In the 19th century most businesses were small, and competitive, independent entrepreneurs flourished. Near the end of the century, however, tendencies toward concentration of economic resources in the form of trusts and consolidations emerged, undermining small businesses. Monopoly capitalism superseded competitive capitalism, and huge firms developed, replacing the independent and the self-employed businessman and businesswoman.

As firms increased in size, a need for foremen, supervisors, and managers to coordinate and control the larger workforce emerged, creating an upper level of white collar workers (Mills, 1951; Braverman, 1974; Stone, 1975; Edwards, 1979). In addition, as corporate firms consolidated their operations under one roof, an army of technical and clerical workers was also required, forming the lower white collar ranks of hierarchical organizations. The expansion in advertising, banking, insurance, and health care fueled the demand for clerks, clerical workers, technicians, and service workers.[2]

The conditions of work for lower-level white collar employees have historically varied, depending on the firm's size, its operations, and the level of labor resistance (Edwards, 1979). According to Richard Edwards, bureaucratic control eventually evolved as a means to control both upper- and lower-level white collar workers in large firms, after a series of other labor control experiments.

Bureaucratic control is an invisible system of control in which workers are manipulated by detailed written rules guiding work tasks, evaluation, and supervision. "Proper behavior," or commitment to the goals of the employer, is fostered and rewarded by "professional privilege." Organizations deem these workers "professional," and imbue them with greater status than nonprofessionals. The purpose is to create a more self-controlled, status-conscious, and divided workforce. Management in the bureaucratic organization succeeds in this endeavor by encouraging educational credentialism and strong identification with the occupation, in the belief that this will decrease the professional's association with nonprofessionals and their tactics, especially the most powerful tactic for defending workers' rights--trade unionism (Edwards, 1979).

Theoretical debates have flourished over definitions of this professional white collar group. Many social scientists disagree with Edwards's interpretation of control within the bureaucratic firm and argue that educated wage-earning professionals are less susceptible to control at work because of their exclusive monopoly over scientifically based skills and knowledge (Friedson, 1973a; Bell, 1973). Others claim, however, that educated wage-earning professionals, because of their dependence on salaried employment within the firm, are instead, "proletarianized," subject to external authority, decreased autonomy, and degradation of status and reward (Derber, 1982, 1983; Larson, 1979, 1980; Oppenheimer, 1985, 1975, 1973; Braverman, 1974).

This debate has permeated discussions of class in the social science literature as well. Theorists argue over the proper conceptualization of the new middle class, a disparate group ranging from clerical workers to college professors (Mills, 1951). While many currently decry the actual disappearance of the middle class due to an ever widening gulf between the rich and the poor in American society (Newman, 1988, 1993; Phillips, 1993),[3] the debate on the constitution of the new middle class raged for several years (Vanneman and Cannon, 1987). According to Mills, this new middle class shared a common fear of falling into the proletariat yet was incapable of autonomous political organization due to its diverse material and psychological interests. Thus Mills, who has been joined by more recent new-middle-class theorists, argued that these workers would follow either business or labor, depending on which proved the stronger (Mills, 1951). They had no inherent loyalties to either but were susceptible to influence and pressure.

Mills's position has been disputed by other theorists who argue that educated wage earners represent a new working class. Educated wage earners, they suggest, like industrial workers, labor for a wage and lack control over their work (Gorz, 1967; Mallet, 1975; Stodder, 1973; Gintis, 1970). Yet adherents of this view point out that the identity of such workers rests not with the working class but in opposition to it. They resist being treated as working class and focus instead on their special privileges--those that separate the credentialed workforce from the blue collar worker (Gorz, 1972).

There are middle positions in this debate as well. Poulantzas (1973, 1975) maintained that educated wage earners are members of the new petite bourgeoisie. Although they do not actually produce commodities, they carry out the ideological and political goals of the dominant sectors of society. Ehrenreich and Ehrenreich suggest this group comprises a separate professional managerial class (PMC), distinct from the working or middle class (Ehrenreich and Ehrenreich, 1979). That is, educated wage earners are part of a new class, with distinct interests and functions, situated between labor and capital. According to these scholars, the PMC shares with all other wage earners the condition of being a salaried employee, subject to external control. At the same time, however, the PMC carries out the managerial function of enforcing social control upon other wage earners and identifies with "progress."

Adding controversy to the debate are proletarianization theorists (Derber, 1983; Larson, 1980; Gorz, 1967; Mallet, 1975; Stodder, 1973; Oppenheimer, 1973; Bellaby and Oribabor, 1977; Aronowitz, 1983) and professionalization theorists (Ehrenreich and Ehrenreich, 1979; Friedson, 1973a, 1970; Bell, 1973; Gorz, 1972; Poulantzas, 1975). The former posit that educated wage earners' dependence on salaried employment in rationalized, profit-making bureaucracies has led to decreased control over the conditions of work, implying a decline in their class position. The professionalization theorists suggest the educated wage earners' monopoly over scientifically based skills in the bureaucratic organization has led to increased control over the conditions of their work, implying an elevation in their class position (Ehrenreich and Ehrenreich, 1979; Friedson, 1973a, 1970; Bell, 1973; Gorz, 1972; Poulantzas, 1975).

Both the professional and the proletarianization perspectives implicitly address the educated wage earners' class position. However, both camps falter when they attempt to portray the subjective dimension of class identity. Their theoretical positions cannot predict whether the new class will identify with organized labor or with individualized forms of social mobility. I suggest that the inability to understand the consciousness of the new class stems from misunderstandings of the actual labor process that governs the work lives of educated, salaried, white collar workers. The analysis of the labor process is insufficiently detailed and does not distinguish between very different segments of the workforce, since workers are often classified by their broad occupational categories, too general to capture the wide variations in the work process.

The resolution of these conceptual problems lies, I suggest, in E. O. Wright's concept of contradictory class locations (Wright, 1976). He argues that class position is a function of a worker's place in the labor process. By examining white collar workers within the structure of production, one discovers that, first, white collar workers are a distinctly heterogeneous group, comprising disparate occupations with varied levels of control in the workplace. Second, within each occupation, there are segments with varied levels of control over their work. Third, and most important, these segments are themselves inherently ambiguous: they have greater levels of control over some aspects of their work and lesser amounts of control over other aspects. Thus, Wright suggests, workers occupy contradictory class locations: some characteristics of their work resemble aspects of blue collar assembly line workers, and some resemble aspects of management.

The study reported in this book employs Wright's theories on class to analyze the objective class position of white collar workers in order to show its value for understanding the nature of class identity. I examine variation in the labor process as it affects one occupation and show how this variation differentiates subgroups within an occupational category. I do not assume, however, that class structure, no matter how accurately defined, necessarily determines class identity and collective action. As Katznelson warns, it is too easy to assume that "'classes-in-themselves' will, indeed, must, 'act-for themselves' at some [magical] moment" (Katznelson, 1986: 6). This study seeks to avoid that pitfall and addresses the interaction of objective class position, subjective thought, and collective action. It does so by comparing the ways in which individuals sharing class positions express their "shared maps of social reality," as Geertz has described it, which coalesce, to form different "autonomous political affiliations" (Geertz, 1964: 63-64). In what ways do workers who share similar objective conditions of work collectively express these shared experiences?

This approach is derived from a body of literature on the anthropology and sociology of work that focuses on the relationship between work and shared cultural meanings, or ideology. Braverman's powerful analysis of the degradation of work (Braverman, 1974) has been widely criticized for its lack of attention to the active role of the worker in this process (Burawoy, 1978). His neglect of the contest between workers and management in the transformation of the 19th-century workplace triggered a plethora of studies focusing on just that: work culture, or various forms of worker resistance, informal relationships on the shop floor and the formation of shared values and symbolic systems in department stores, offices, hospitals, and shop floors (Burawoy, 1979; Melosh, 1982; Lamphere, 1985, 1986; Benson, 1984; Shapiro-Perl, 1984; Sacks, 1984, 1988). Some authors focus on the way in which cultural norms and networks forged in the family are later brought into the workplace, shaping behaviors and forms of resistance at work (Gutman, 1976; Hareven, 1982; Hareven and Vinovskis, 1975; Lamphere, 1985, 1986; Sacks, 1984). Others focus on the historical dimensions of cultural norms themselves, which shape different cohorts' "symbolic dialects," or varied interpretations of the same event (Newman, 1986, 1987; Wilentz, 1983).

It is essential to see work culture as a "complex set of relationships [in the workplace] between cultural meaning or ideology on the one hand and behavioral strategies or practice on the other" (Lamphere, 1985: 521; Benson, 1984; Shapiro-Perl, 1984). I have attempted to understand such cultural meanings and behavioral strategies in relation to class position.

My focus does not negate the importance of studies that suggest factors outside the workplace, such as place of residence, have a major influence on workers' politics (Halle, 1984; Gans, 1988). I simply contend that "professionals'" class identity can best be understood by examining their work culture, or the relation between ideology and collective action in conjunction with a focus on the labor process.

I have wed these approaches through a case study of nursing, a small segment of the white collar workforce, has historically embodied the contradictions of control and subordination, of autonomy and dependence, and varied forms of collective action. Two out of three nurses are employed in hospitals (Bureau of Labor Statistics, 1992), paradigm cases of organizations that approximate the conditions of work that Edwards labels bureaucratic control. In most hospitals, nurses are subject to detailed, written rules governing their work and behavior. In return for their compliance with the goals of management, they are promised "professional privilege"--some form of control over their work and social and economic status.

Nurses have responded to management's policy of bureaucratic control in the workplace with three different strategies: trade unionism, professionalization, and professional unionism. Each reflects a distinctive consciousness or "shared map of social reality." The varied cultural meanings suggest that nursing is a divided profession; different nursing groups are embedded in different labor processes, influencing their varied perceptions of both problems and solutions in the workplace.

To understand this diversity of groups within the nursing occupation, whose actual class position varies according to the roles they perform within the system of medical production, I employ E. O. Wright's concept of contradictory class locations to ascertain nurses' specific class positions. To determine nurses' differential class identities, I focus on their choice of collective action (trade unionism, professional unionism, or professionalization) and their interpretations of the concept of professionalism.

THE CASE OF NURSING

Prior to World War II, American nurses depended primarily on private duty for employment, caring for single patients in their homes (Melosh, 1982; Mottus, 1980; Reverby, 1982). They often suffered from 24-hour workdays and seasonal employment patterns, finding more work in the winter than the summer months. Nevertheless, private duty nurses had minimal supervision and exercised a certain degree of control over their conditions of work.

Since the end of World War II, nurses have been employed primarily in hospitals. As in other industries, scientific management techniques have permeated hospital work. Following Frederick Taylor's scientific management approach (Taylor, 1947), hospitals have reduced tasks to their component parts, enforced sharp divisions of labor, and minimized employee control of working conditions (Ehrenreich and Ehrenreich, 1976; Kotelchuck, 1976; C. Brown, 1973; Reverby and Rosner, 1979; Reverby, 1982).

The rapid growth of medical technology in the late 1940s resulted in the creation of nursing specialties, paralleling the development of physicians' specialties (such as cardiac, pulmonary, and intensive care). But as doctors gained status, nurses lost status and autonomy as hospital employees, which they had previously enjoyed in private, albeit precarious, positions. Often each nurse now performed only one task. Perhaps most degrading was team nursing: a team of nurses, each having a specific task, would travel around a unit or the entire hospital, providing a specific form of care, such as inserting IVs.

Many hospitals gave up this more Taylorized form of nursing work and replaced it with a system of primary nursing, with each nurse responsible for all aspects of care for a given number of patients. Although this form of nursing work is less Taylorized, it has intensified nursing work since fewer, more educated, nurses are employed. As a result of this speed-up, in which fewer nurses do the work that was previously performed by greater numbers of less skilled workers, such as practical nurses, aides, and technicians, greater pressure is exerted on those who remain. Nursing has lost many of its traditional skills to other emerging occupations such as x-ray, physical therapy, respiratory therapy, pharmacy, and social work (Wagner, 1980; also see Table 3.2). Some fear this de-skilling threatens the very existence of nursing as an occupation.

How has nursing, this white collar professional workforce, responded to such changes in work conditions? Nurses have tried three collective strategies since the late 19th century--trade unionism, professional unionism, and professionaliza-tion--each worth looking at. The professionalization project was initiated in the 1890s by nursing educators and administrators (Reverby, 1982) in an attempt to gain control over the supply and demand in their occupation. By decreasing the supply and mandating higher educational credentials, they hoped to increase the demand and, hopefully, their economic reward. This strategy, which has continued to the present day and promises to continue into the 21st century, focuses on political struggle outside the workplace, between occupations, to achieve their goals within the workplace. Nursing administrators have lobbied state and federal government officials for full control over the licensure process for nursing. They have sought to attain control over their own educational process, occupational turf, and the number and type of nursing practitioners. Thus, the aim of professionalization is monopoly control over the occupation, along the lines of the medical model (Larson, 1977).

Trade unionism is a different collective response that has been employed primarily by nonadministrative, nonmanagerial nurses, initiated in 1910. Its focus is economic struggle within the workplace between management and labor, using such tactics as collective bargaining and work stoppage (strikes, mass resignations, and sick-outs). The aim of trade unionism is to attain greater benefits from, and control over, conditions of work such as staff-patient ratios, job security, salary, and autonomy.

Finally, professional unionism is an approach that was initiated by the American Nurses Association (ANA) in 1946 in an attempt to deflect nursing membership from trade unions. In some respects, professional unionism is a fusion of the other two strategies in that it combines a collective bargaining approach as well as a professionalization strategy. The ANA imbued its state affiliates with the power to bargain collectively with employers, and they do engage in minimal work stoppages.[4] But they also focus much of their energy on lobbying state legislatures for monopoly control over the occupation. This dual focus derives from the structure of the professional union. It is embedded within the state professional associations as simply another department within the association. Thus, the professional unions are subordinate to the overall goals of the state professional associations which are members of the larger national professional association (the ANA). It is an approach favored most consistently by middle managerial nurses, some of whom are and some of whom are not eligible for membership in its bargaining unit.

OBJECTIVES AND HYPOTHESIS OF STUDY

To examine the relationship of nurses' collective response to their conditions of work, nurses' position in the labor process, and class identity, this study poses one central question: does nurses' class position, determined by their location in the structure of production, using Wright's notion of contradictory class locations, have a determining effect on their class identity indicated by choice of collective strategy (trade unionism, professional unionism, or professionalization)? The findings of this study suggest that Wright's view is insufficient by itself. While it is true that class location is a significant force in creating an ideology of interests, so too is a differential interpretation of professionalism.

Class position is understood in terms of the framework developed by E. O. Wright (1976, 1980) who defines class entirely in terms of control relations.[5] He divides control into three realms: economic, political, and ideological. Economic control refers to control over what is produced in the workplace and what is done with the profits from the process of accumulation. Political control refers to control within the supervisory hierarchy. Ideological control refers to control over conception and execution within production. In keeping with these parameters, the class position of nurses in this study is contradictory. That is, they possess some characteristics reminiscent of the proletariat since they lack control over many aspects of their work. At the same time, they resemble the bourgeoisie since they have considerable control over other aspects of their work. Given these contradictions inherent in their labor processes, the question is, with which group do they ultimately identify: management or labor?

Nurses with the least amount of economic, political, and ideological control occupy a low class position. Those with greater but not full amounts of control in each arena occupy a medium class position, the most contradictory of all class locations. Those with the greatest amounts of control in each domain are those located in a high class position. Nurses' job description (staff, middle manager, or administrative nurse) is used as an indicator of position within the labor process.

Nurses' diverse experience in the workplace also produces three disparate interpretations of professionalism, an all-pervasive construct in the culture of nursing and white collar work in general. Since professionalism has been imposed from above (by hospital management and nursing educational institutions), it is subject to varied interpretations by those below. I suggest, in fact, that these varied interpretations draw from different strands in American culture itself.

The oldest interpretation of professionalism reflects the larger cultural construct of free market individualism, or capitalist individualism, a term coined by Herbert Gans (1988) that refers to individuals who seek social mobility by maximizing their profits through pursuit of market control, risk taking, and adherence to the principles of meritocracy. Underlying this free market vision of professionalism are also the wholesome attributes of the professional: competence, autonomy, and altruism. According to this vision, those individuals who enhance their human capital and succeed in gaining market control are worthy of attaining professional privilege--a privilege ultimately translated into social and economic reward.

The second interpretation of professionalism draws on the American tradition of collectivism, as employed by trade unions. Nurses with this perception of professionalism understand it to mean having enough collective work control over such work conditions as autonomy, job security, and work shift, enabling quality performance on the job, deemed a virtuous activity.

Finally, the last interpretation of professionalism is a composite of the former two, combining both perceptions of work control and individualism. This form of individualism, which Gans termed "popular individualism" (Gans, 1988), is more a personal flight from workplace constraints than an overt pursuit of individual profit maximization and power. Also believing in the culture of meritocracy, this vision of professionalism involves a belief in credentialism and compliant behaviors to achieve greater status and control in the workplace.

A survey of what nurses actually think shows a high correlation between class position, choice of collective strategy, and interpretation of professionalism. Eighty percent of the nurses in a high class location interpret professionalism according to the capitalist individualism approach, and 60 percent of these nurses support the collective strategy of professionalization (monopoly control over nursing education and labor markets through legislative mandate) to attain their vision. Both this perception of professionalism and this choice of organizational strategy are indicative of a managerial identity.[6]

Eighty-four percent of the nurses in a low class position interpret professionalism to mean work control--collective control over such conditions of work as autonomy, job security, salary, promotions, and the like. Sixty percent of the nurses in this class position support trade unionism: collective, economic struggle in the workplace between management and employees. Their interpretation of professionalism and their choice of strategy are indicators of a more class-conscious, working class identity.

Seventy-six percent of the nurses in the medium class position translate professionalism to mean a composite of both work control and popular individualism: both collective control over conditions of their work and individualized credentialism and compliant behavior. This more contradictory vision of professionalism is in concert with their more contradictory class location. They carry out both managerial and staff duties yet are subordinate to an array of medical, nursing, and administrative layers above themselves. The strategy that 94 percent of these nurses support is professional unionism, which reflects their ambiguous position of being simultaneously staff and management. Yet they strive for the professional privilege of management: social and economic status. Their more conflictual strategy and vision of professionalism indicates a more contradictory class identity as well: between the workingclass and management, albeit closer to the latter. (See Table 1.1)

METHOD AND BACKGROUND ON RESEARCH SITES

I interviewed all types of nurses at two hospitals in New York City, using an open-ended survey instrument as a guide. (See Appendix A.)[7] Each interview with nurses from the two hospitals lasted for approximately one to three and a half hours and took place in their homes, on the hospital units, in coffee shops, and restaurants, or wherever else we could find a place for private conversation. The sample was constructed via the snowball method. The first individual was located by a letter she had written to *Nurses' Network,* an independent nursing journal committed to changing conditions of nursing work. Once she agreed to participate in the study, she suggested names of other nurses employed at different hospitals. Two locations were finally chosen because the nurses were undergoing change in their collective representatives. Altogether 65 interviews were completed.

Although I made several attempts to engage in participant-observation and "hang out" on the nursing floors for extended periods of time, I was unable to gain official access to any hospital, preventing such participant-observation.[8] I was thus prohibited from witnessing on a daily basis the varied nursing labor processes. The method I used, in-depth interview, did enable discovery of subtle qualitative relationships, such as that between the meaning of professionalism and class identity.

Although this sample is relatively small and the study is located in one of the geographic areas that is more conducive to unionism for nurses (the Northeast), a larger, more representative sample analyzed quantitatively would not necessarily have added to the particular insights revealed here. (For example, the finding that class position within an occupation is highly correlated with a particular world-

TABLE 1.1
Class Position, Choice of Collective Strategy, and Interpretation of Professionalism

Class Position	Collective Strategy	Stated Reason for Choice of Strategy	Definition of Professionalism
Low class position			
TOTAL: 44	Trade Unionism (60%)	Work Conditions (60%)	Work Control (84%)
	Prof. Unionism (34%)	Work Conditions (20%)	Work Control (11%)
		Work Conditions & Prestige (11%)	Popular Individualist (5%)
	Trade or Prof. Union (6%)	Work Conditions (4%)	
		Prestige (5%)	
Medium class position			
TOTAL: 17	Trade Unionism (6%)	Work Conditions (6%)	Work Control (24%)
	Prof. Unionism (94%)	Work Conditions & Status (12%)	Work Control & Popular Ind. (76%)
		Work Conditions Prestige & Credentialism (41%)	
		Prestige (41%)	
High class position			
TOTAL: 5	Professionalization (60%)	Prestige, Power, & Credentialism (100%)	Capitalist Individualist (80%)
	Prof. Union (40%)		Popular Ind. & Worker Control (20%)

view, transcending an overall occupational vantage point, may be obscured by a statistical study of, for example, trade union membership among nurses.)[9]

The case study method utilized in this analysis also brought out another confounding finding: that the collective organization compatible with the worldview of nurses in a low class position may be unavailable to them. Low trade union membership among nurses in a low class position may have as much, if not more, to do with the quality of available trade unions as it does with any adherence to an anti-union ideology. The nurses in a low class position at one of the hospitals in this study believe in the ideology of trade unionism, particularly revealed in their work control vision of professionalism, but found themselves in the unenviable position of having to decertify their bargaining representative due to the deterioration of Local 1199 of the Retail, Wholesale and Department Store Trade Union (RWDSU), during 1983-84. The nurses in a low class position at the other hospital, however, found their efforts to bring in a trade union opposed and squelched by the sophisticated anti-union techniques of their management. Hence, context and history matter. They do not determine a group's ambitions but may well influence strategy and/or the ultimate gap between ambitions and reality.

In sum, the case study method utilized was chosen partially by default but mostly because of its advantages in unraveling the subtleties of relationships between class position and class identity. Moreover, it provided a lucid view of workplace ideologies in formation.

RESEARCH SITES

The research sites were chosen because nurses at each location had been in the throes of debate over their choice of collective labor strategy. At one site, which I call St. John's Hospital (a pseudonym to protect the identity of the nurses), had decertified their trade union in 1984 (the League of Registered Nurses, Local 1199 of RWDSU). At the other site, which I call Mt. Zion Hospital, nurses had recently attempted to decertify the professional union in 1982 (New York State Nurses' Association-NYSNA) although the attempt was unsuccessful.

Mt. Zion (also a pseudonym), is a large non-government, nonprofit, short-term (voluntary hospital) medical center located in New York City. It is replete with the most recent advances in medical technology, specialization, and labor management. Patients come from far and wide to receive care at Mt. Zion and often serve as teaching tools for residents and interns. It has 1065 beds and a patient census of 946 (the average number of patients per day receiving care over a 12-month period). The total number of personnel (full-time equivalents, FTEs) at Mt. Zion is 5064.

St. John's Hospital is a smaller teaching hospital located in Brooklyn. It is defined as a nongovernment, nonprofit, short-term (voluntary) hospital, which is characterized by less advanced medical technology, specialization, and labor management. It serves primarily patients from the local community and is one of the affiliated hospitals for clinical teaching with the State University of New York (along with seven other hospitals). It has 567 beds, a patient census of 501, and a total of 2554 FTE personnel (AHA Guide to Health Care Field; 1989: A212).

General History of Research Sites

The historic development of both hospitals follows the general principles delineated by Richard Brown in his analysis of the role that philanthropists played in shaping modern hospitals and medicine (R. Brown, 1979: Ch. 5). Between 1890 and 1925 medical science was transformed from a gentleman's occupation to a powerful scientific and technical force in American society. Brown suggests that corporate magnates of this era were committed to pragmatic forms of education that would prove useful to industry and the general economy. They embraced the notion of technological medicine because it provided them with a compatible worldview that focused on disease within the body, as opposed to various forms of industrial or occupational disease.

Major foundations formed a General Education Board and played a central role in shaping medical education. They sought a rationalized health care system directed by medical schools that were committed to a scientific and technological type of medicine. The board's goals included the creation of well-equipped medical centers, where training, research, and clinical practice would take place. Hospitals were to be the prospective center point of this system and therefore became ardent advocates of the philanthropists' goals.

In 1927 the philanthropists had formed the Committee on the Costs of Medical Care, whose members included such giants as Rockefeller, Rosenwald, Macy, Milbank, and Carnegie and their foundations. They wrote report after report recommending changes in the organization of medical care. By 1946, this group had been joined by hospital administrators, health insurance leaders, and even the American Medical Association (AMA), in a loose coalition that won the passage of the Hill-Burton Act. This brought federal dollars into the picture: $5 billion for hospital construction and modernization.

After World War II, the federal government began taking over the philanthropists' role in financing reforms in medical education and, later, in the operating costs of medical schools and hospitals. By the 1950s there was a growing public concern about a doctor shortage (supported and promoted by the AMA), and Congress began to approve more construction grants and traineeships for medical schools. In addition, medical research dollars from the National Institutes of Health began flowing generously.

By the mid-1960s, Medicare (a social security program covering most medical services for Americans over age 65) and Medicaid (a welfare-linked program for the medically indigent) bills were passed over the medical profession's vehement protests. Suddenly these two programs became a bottomless money pit for hospitals, construction companies, banks, medical supply industries, and physicians. Hospital and doctor fees rose astronomically because insured patients retained minimal financial responsibility for their own bills. Medicare and Medicaid, along with private health insurance, effectively subsidized the expansion of high-tech medical care. Hospitals felt confident that everything would be covered: from automated blood-chemistry analysis machines (costing upwards of $100,000), to computerized axial tomography (CAT) scanners (costing $300,000 to $750,000) (R. Brown, 1979: 203). Expensive technology spread like wildfire until the 1990s, virtually unchecked by considerations of cost. An AMA study underscores this point. It found that in 1989, on a per capita basis, the United States had four times as many magnetic resonance imaging (MRI) machines (at $1000 a scan) as Germany and eight times as many as Canada (Eckholm, 1993: 70).

Thus, federal and state government took over where the private foundations left off in supporting the explosion in medical care costs. In the mid-1970s sixty cents of every dollar spent by medical schools was provided by the federal government (R. Brown, 1979: 227). By 1992, 9 percent of all federal spending (compared to military spending, comprising 22 percent) went to Medicare costs, in large part due to a dramatic rise in the volume of physicians' services to Medicare patients. Critics argue that over one-quarter of these services are of questionable value, provided basically to line physicians' pockets. The chairman of the Department of Medicine at Georgetown University says, "Ten percent of [these] physician services [are] of no real value to the patient [and] . . . perhaps 25% are of some small value to the patient" (Eckholm 1993:23). Corporate interests in the insurance, drug, medical supply, and construction industries, along with a new echelon of health care administrators, planners, and physicians, have been in their heyday.

In the 1980s, a damper was placed on the health care orgy. The Congressional Budget Office projected that Medicare would run out of money by 1988, and in response, Congress passed legislation in 1982 requiring the Department of Health and Human Services to find a way to curb reimbursements (Gilbert, 1990: 23). The department adopted a system of diagnostic-related groups (DRGs), in which 487 categories of illness were established, each assigned a fixed fee although fees vary by region (rural versus urban hospitals). By 1983 the Department of Health and Human Services began implementing the DRG system for all in-hospital services to Medicare recipients. Fee for service is still applied to outpatient care and doctors' visits.

A parallel system, the resource-based relative value scale (RBRVS), is being phased in for physicians as well. This system divides Medicare treatments into 7,000 categories, according to the time and expertise required. The more valuable the procedure is to the patient and the more time it takes to perform the procedure, the more Medicare will pay (Eckholm, 1993). The DRG system has achieved its goal of cutting costs to some degree. The rate of increase in Medicare outlays declined from 19 percent in 1981-82 to 4 percent in 1987-88 (Gilbert, 1990: 30). Nevertheless, this system has brought about its own negative side effects. Patients are often discharged before they are capable of functioning on their own; exorbitant, uninsured home health care costs are incurred by individuals; and patients are denied medical tests and procedures because they are now less profitable for the hospital. To deal with the spiraling costs of medical care, policy makers have reached a feverish pitch, competing to hammer out their own vision of the financial future for the American health care system. The battle between proponents of national health insurance, where the federal government alone would pay for all citizens' health care costs, and managed competition, seems to be weighted heavily toward the latter; nevertheless, the political economic future of American health care has yet to be completely determined.

Mt. Zion Hospital

Mt. Zion Hospital was, like other voluntary hospitals, created by well-respected members of the local community who believed that the "deserving poor" should have access to some facility for their health and welfare. Although voluntary institutions were initially established to provide free public services, they were firmly controlled by the private philanthropists who funded them. In addition, most voluntary hospitals were founded to serve special ethnic or religious groups, and patients who were of another faith, contagious, or morally suspect were not welcome (Annual Report, 1986).

Mt. Zion was originally known as the Jews hospital, founded in 1855 by prominent German Jewish philanthropists who intended their hospital to serve Jews. The onset of the American Civil War changed the patient population at Jews' Hospital when a soldiers' ward was established, and individuals of all faiths were finally accepted, as well as those with contagious diseases such as typhoid, who were previously screened out. Severe overcrowding in the tenement houses of New York City, child labor, prostitution, and generally unsanitary conditions during this period also contributed to the altered patient population. In 1866 the name was changed from the Jews' Hospital to Mt. Zion Hospital. The location changed as well, from 28th Street, which was surrounded by tomato crops and dirt roads, to uptown, where the air was "more pure" and the atmosphere more tranquil (Hirsch and Dougherty, 1952:48).

Wealthy wives of the hospital trustees, physicians, and others involved in the affairs of the hospital developed a Ladies Auxiliary Society in 1868 to assist in furnishing Mt. Zion's "inmates" with clothing and other necessities. They initiated charitable social functions as a means of raising money for the hospital and were instrumental in professionalizing the occupation of nursing at Mt. Zion. They convinced their husbands of the need for a school of nursing, which would train only respectable, middle-class Jewish women: to replace the poor women who generally occupied these positions. The school was incorporated, with its own board of directors, in 1895. The Ladies Auxiliary Society made every attempt to "impress upon eligible Jewesses the advantages offered by the School." Their duties included the "best practical methods of supplying fresh air . . . disinfecting utensils; reporting to the physicians on the state of excretions, expectoration, pulse, skin, temperature, intelligence, delirium, eruptions, formation of matter and other general care taking areas" (Hirsch and Dougherty, 1952:69).

By 1902 Mt. Zion marked its fiftieth anniversary with a move to its third and final location even farther uptown in Manhattan. The names on the buildings read like a roster of the philanthropists who organized the structure of the medical center (Brown, 1979). Adolph Lewisohn, a trustee from 1889 to 1938, was responsible for financing medical laboratories and their expansions throughout that period. The Guggenheims were major contributors responsible for the early hospital expansion, as the Guggenheim Pavilion attests, built in 1910. Henry Einstein gave money for a Children's Pavilion in 1921, now called the Einstein-Falk Pavilion. Other major donors Stella Housman and Florence and William Walter (Annual Report, 1976: 12). Based on such funding, a continuous process of expansion and improvement of the physical plant has taken place since 1904, with a hiatus only during the Great Depression.

A new complex was built, more than twice the size of its predecessor, with 432 beds in four different pavilions: a Surgical Pavilion, a Medical Pavilion, a Central Administration Building (which also housed a 200-seat synagogue), a Children's Pavilion, and a 53-bed Private Pavilion, among others (Annual Report 1976: 11).

Medical specialization grew at a rapid pace during this period as well, especially given the orientation of the philanthropists: away from the general "art" of medicine, toward science and technology. In 1900 Mt. Zion purchased its first x-ray machine and developed its first Radiology Department. The surgical service was reorganized into specialized areas of genitourinary, neurosurgery, surgery of the neck and face, and surgery of the abdomen. In 1907, the first Fellowship Program in Pathology was established in the name of its donor, George Blumenthal. From 1923 onward, donors established several fellowships in different specialties, which were the precursors to a formal clinical postgraduate center at the hospital. Thus, the link between philanthropists' interests and the direction of medical specialization is clear (Annual Report, 1976).

Between 1927 and World War II, expansion of the facilities came to a standstill. The depression put a damper on the contributions of several of the philanthropists. But by the early 1950s building picked up once again, with the Hill-Burton Act, which availed hospitals of federal funds for capital projects. Federal dollars for research increased as well, and Mt. Zion ranked twenty-seventh among all institutions receiving research grant dollars from the National Institutes of Health (Annual Report, 1989: 356). The hospital's residency program more than doubled, from 26 residents in 1942 to 114, and 25 full-time postgraduate students in 1945. By 1962, the hospital's priorities were redirected toward establishing a new School of Medicine and Medical Center. The philosophic underpinnings of the new medical school were in accord with the original outline devised by the Committee on the Costs of Medical Care in 1927: emphasizing strong basic sciences.

Twenty-six million dollars for the new medical complex came from the U.S. Public Health Service. By 1971 federal funding for research, financial aid, and building began drying up (partially due to the Vietnam War, which was soaking up federal tax dollars), and Mt. Zion ran a deficit. Fewer teaching faculty were hired. In response, hospital administrators sought private funds once again for their new building plans. By the 1980s, with the onset of DRGs, hospitals became even more costconscious, and Mt. Zion began cutting back on all nonmedical staff, reducing the number of patient-days, beds, and diagnostic tests. In sum, Mt. Zion, a capital-intensive, major research and teaching hospital, which has historically had heavy philanthropic support, became increasingly vulnerable to public cuts and funding.

St. John's Hospital

The early history of St. John's Hospital is similar to Mt. Zion's but is also closely linked to the history of Brooklyn, where it is situated. In 1856 Brooklyn was the third largest city in the United States, with a population of 200,000. Its chief industries were shipping, manufacturing, and the distillation of whisky. The majority of Brooklyn's population were newly arrived immigrants from Germany and Ireland, and poverty and overcrowding were common conditions. Homeless children were frequently found roaming the streets along with cows, goats, and pigs. Sanitation was a serious problem, given that there was no municipal water supply and individuals were forced to obtain their water from backyard wells or public cisterns (Donaldson, 1933: Ch. 1).

The total number of deaths during 1856 was calculated at 3762, due to diseases such as cholera, dysentery, scarlet fever, and tuberculosis. There was only one hospital in Brooklyn at this time, Brooklyn City Hospital. Most individuals with any financial means avoided it, choosing care in their homes instead. Victims of industrial or street accidents were often carried to police stations or drugstores for emergency treatment by an available doctor and then taken home, where the kitchen table would serve as an operating table. Only if patients were poor, homeless, or in need of extreme emergency care would they be taken to the hospital (Donaldson, 1933:81).

In 1856 a German physician opened up a free dispensary for the German-speaking poor in Brooklyn. Although the founder of the dispensary, which later became St. John's Hospital, intended to serve only Germans, the great influx of Irish into Brooklyn made this more difficult, and, by 1858 the charitable hospital was officially opened to both Irish and Germans.

The hospital was the first in this country to combine a medical college with a hospital, a concept that was brought back to the United States by physicians who had been studying in Europe in the 1850s. The hospital was initially housed in a private mansion donated by the Perry Estate, located in the Heights section of Brooklyn. This building, with a few additional wings built later on, housed both the early St. John's Hospital and the medical school. In 1859, the hospital suffered acute financial difficulties and was closed down for a year. To save the hospital, the staff physicians, agreed to rely only on their private practice for income until the hospital had regained its solvency. It was reopened when Dr. Dudley, one of the independently wealthy staff physicians, finally purchased the property. Nevertheless, during the Civil War, the hospital went deep into debt once again and, like Mt. Zion Hospital, relied on wounded soldiers for income. These patients, in combination with contributions from wealthy Brooklynites, enabled the hospital to creep out of debt (Winfield, 1915:316). By 1883 the Hoagland Lab was built, across the street from the Perry Mansion, funded by physician and entrepreneur Dr. Cornelius Hoagland. Additional funds were forthcoming when the U.S. War Department chose St. John's as one of the hospitals to care for the wounded from the Spanish-American War.

During this time the hospital developed another new source of income: immigrants who had landed at Ellis Island. The hospital had garnered a contract with the federal government to receive and treat sick newcomers to New York Island. They set up a clinic in the new Ellis Island Hospital, and both the clinic and St. John's Hospital were paid 90 cents a head for adults and 40 cents per child.

St. John's Hospital began to increase its endowments and by 1898, the Polhemus Memorial Clinic was built, funded by Mrs. Polhemus, in memory of her husband, a former regent of St. John's. In 1899, another regent announced he would fund the construction of an entirely new hospital in memory of his brother, Dr. Dudley, the physician who had previously saved it from financial ruin.

Despite these physical plant improvements, by this time other, more successful hospitals had affiliated with established universities with large endowments, where full-time teaching faculty replaced clinical practitioners as teachers. St. John's Hospital was scrutinized by the philanthropists seeking to control the direction of medical education and was criticized in 1910 by the famous Flexner Report. It was said to lack full-time teachers, lab space, adequate clinical facilities, a library, and attention to the basic sciences in its curriculum. (The Flexner Report was a highly influential report commissioned by the Carnegie Foundation to make a full-scale investigation on the status of American hospitals and medical schools.) In an effort to redress its shortcomings, St. John's Medical College separated from the hospital in 1930.

By 1950 the College of Medicine ended its status as a private institution, and under a mandate from the New York state legislature, it merged with the State University of New York, located in another section of Brooklyn. St. John's

Hospital became merely one of seven affiliates of Downstate Medical Center, where clinical teaching is carried on.

Throughout the 1960s, the underpinning of hospital financing had shifted away from philanthropic contributions toward state and federal funds. However, unlike Mt. Zion, St. John's Hospital never developed into a huge medical center and was not a repository for vast sums of federal research or construction dollars. It remained a small affiliate of a state hospital center that received government funds directly. Downstate Medical Center's faculty tripled its size during the 1950s, constructed new buildings, and purchased more up-to-date equipment. St. John's physical plant was improved, but primarily from private dollars, with comparatively minor renovations. During the 1970s Fuller contributed funds and built an extension, housing general patients in the Fuller Pavilion. In 1983, the Pollack Pavilion was completed, housing such units as the intensive care unit (ICU), critical care unit (CCU), and obstetrics-gynecology (ObGyn) unit, as well as operating rooms. In 1989, the Othmer Building was completed, which houses doctors' offices, the dental clinic, and such departments as Radiation.

HOSPITAL WORKFORCE

Despite the differences between the two hospitals, Mt. Zion, as a major, world-renowned medical center, and St. John's, as a small affiliate of a state medical center, national financial expansions and contractions in the health care picture are similarly reflected in the organization of hospital work at both hospitals. Such economic fluctuations weigh heavily on changes in their workforces, ultimately reflected in the varied forms of labor organization as well.

After World War II, the hospitals chose to hire a primarily cheap, unskilled, nonmedical workforce. In New York City hospitals, for example, twice as many nurses' aides and practical nurses were hired as registered nurses. (See Table 3.2.) When funds were directed more toward increased medical specialization and technological advances, new, specialized nonphysician health care workers were hired at both Mt. Zion and St. John's.

Initially, all types of nurses, such as aides, licensed practical nurses (LPNs) and registered nurses (RNs), carried out the duties connected to high-tech medicine as the need arose, such as respiratory therapy or chemotherapy preparation. However, this changed as nursing and physician shortages occurred in the 1960s, brought on by the professional associations themselves (Larson, 1977; Backup and Molinaro, 1984) to upgrade their social and economic status. As a result of the artificially created shortage, the AMA and the American Hospital Association fostered the development of newer, cheaper assistants, technicians, and technologists (e.g., respiratory therapists, medical technologists, physicians' assistants), to relieve both shortages and to pick up the new specialties, without medicine's loss of control over the health care system (Backup and Molinero, 1984: 202). Hence, as respondents at both Mt. Zion and St. John's concur, various less expensive, salaried technicians emerged, such as electromyographic technicians, pharmacy technicians, and radiation therapy technicians, taking over tasks that were previously performed by nurses.

This form of cost cutting also resulted in increased interest in unionization. At Mt. Zion in 1959, 800 workers boycotted the hospital's cafeteria in a lunch hour demonstration, demanding that the hospital recognize their chosen union: Local 1199. Those on the bottom of the hospital hierarchy--dietary, laundry, and housekeeping workers--were the first group who most desired union organization. The LPNs, aides, and orderlies were slightly less susceptible to unionism initially. RNs were even less interested, perhaps because their work was more isolated, as they spent time alone with patients (Fink and Greenberg, 1989:49).[10] Nevertheless, by 1964, Local 1199 alone had organized 21,000 white collar hospital workers (Fink and Greenberg, 1989: 116).

Until the mid-1970s, hospitals had less of a pressing incentive to control costs by cutting staff. They wanted inexpensive labor but more of it. Health care providers were able to afford this because they were in a system where the higher their charges were, the higher were their reimbursements from third-party payers, including increased labor costs. In the late 1970s, however, financial restraints were imposed on hospitals by government. The health care environment had changed, and hospital administrators had a greater incentive to cut back on staff. During this period, the vice president of personnel at Mt. Zion characterized the hospital as "an altogether different industry, one that is laying off, that is competitive, [and] . . . sensitive to the costs of having a union on its premises (Fink and Greenberg, 1989: 179). The administrative strategy changed to one where less skilled workers were laid off, and fewer, more highly trained workers were hired. As one nursing administrator from St. John's put it in 1985, this would enable hospitals to "get a bigger bang for their buck." Administrators assumed they could squeeze greater productivity out of a smaller but more highly trained workforce at lower cost.

Nursing professionalizers and hospital administrators found common ground during this period, joining forces to hire more highly educated nurses with bachelor of science and even master of nursing degrees. The less skilled, licensed practical nurses and nurses' aides were laid off. The result of this strategy, however, was tremendous "reality shock," as the nurses describe it, for the college-educated nurses were trained in nursing theory, not practice. In addition, these nurses were not necessarily more highly skilled but rather more highly educated, and they suffered from overwork, as anyone would, as ancillary personnel were let go. As a result, registered nurses became more susceptible to unionism and a primary target for union organizers: their numbers increased by 13 percent in New York City hospitals between 1975 and 1980, while total FTE personnel dropped by 6.5 percent (Fink and Greenberg, 1989: 169).

Nursing Unionism at Mt. Zion

Registered nurses at Mt. Zion experienced these trends. By the early 1980s, they were overworked and had lost control over conditions of their work. They lived with mandatory overtime, few weekends off, poor staff-patient ratios, continual shift rotations, inadequate pay, and 26 percent annual rent increases in their hospital-owned apartments. Both nursing supervisors and staff nurses had been represented by the NYSNA since 1970 (Annual Report, 1970: 156). Local 1199 won representation of licensed practical nurses and aides shortly thereafter but had already won their hearts and minds by 1959, during the major strike against the hospital for union recognition, which they lost (Fink and Greenberg, 1989: 70).

On September 10, 1982, after several years of growing dissatisfaction with NYSNA, the elected body of 10 registered nurses, comprising the Executive Committee of the Mt. Zion Council of Nursing Practitioners, voted to recommend that registered nurses decertify their professional nurses' association, NYSNA. The watershed issue occurred in 1979, after their contract had expired and NYSNA had negotiated a contract that the members did not even know was imminent. The Mt. Zion nurses felt NYSNA had no idea what the nurses wanted in a contract and that it collaborated with management just to get one signed. The members rejected the contract. NYSNA then encouraged the nurses to vote for a strike, which they did, with a vote of 1200 to 28 in favor of striking. When the nurses were ready to walk, NYSNA pulled out its support. The hospital proceeded to force the association to court over the strike for failing to file a strike notice. NYSNA continued to fail Mt. Zion nurses on several counts. It provided Mt. Zion nurses with an inexperienced attorney, whereas the hospital was equipped with a lawyer from one of the most prestigious firms in New York. The lawyer representing the nurses did not even agree with the association's position. In addition, without the knowledge or consent of the negotiating team, NYNSA,[11] in concert with management, had chosen an arbitrator to settle the contract dispute. During the arbitration, the Mt. Zion RNs had to pull the association's lawyer out and correct his presentation of their case themselves.

When the hospital reopened the nurses' contract several months later, NYSNA (still their representative) left the Executive Committee of Mt. Zion nurses without any legal or financial support. Management went to the table with seven vice presidents; the nurses had only themselves. All grievances, from changes in the absenteeism policy to salary increases, were handled by the Executive Committee now.

NYSNA had assigned four different representatives to Mt. Zion in four years, two of whom were brand new to the job. They were assigned to represent not only 1500 Mt. Zion nurses but over 1000 RNs at Columbia Presbyterian Hospital and RNs from several other institutions in New York City as well. To top it off, Mt. Zion nurses claimed their representatives were never available, neither answering telephone calls nor appearing on the premises.

Most important, Mt. Zion nurses argued that NYSNA perpetuated an inherent conflict of interest within the professional union. The nursing administrators, members of hospital management, were simultaneously members of NYSNA, the bargaining agent for staff nurses. Thus, management voted, along with staff nurses, on general and economic welfare (union) issues in NYSNA (Archives, letter from the Council of Nursing Practitioners to Colleagues, 1982).

Nurses at Mt. Zion, fed up with the misrepresentations and what they saw as leadership of dubious loyalty, attempted to decertify NYSNA. They were courted by the Federation of Nurses/United Federation of Teachers, and the League of Registered Nurses, Local 1199, in addition to NYSNA. A protracted battle ensued from September through November between management and Mt. Zion staff nurses. First and foremost management wanted no union at all and sent letters to the staff encouraging them to vote for this position. (Unionism was, in fact, nowhere on the ballot.) Management's second choice was NYSNA, and the director of nursing sent letters to the rank and file with not-so-subtle hints encouraging their vote for an organization that "maintains the highest standards of professional nursing care and practice," the slogan NYSNA used in its campaign. In addition, the nursing administration used intimidation tactics on newly recruited Filipino nurses, with threats that they would lose their H-1 visas (temporary work permit) if they decertified NYSNA. Other union-busting techniques were employed as well, such as closely watching the staff, auditing their every move, and inhibiting organizing activities, by, for example, docking pay from nurses who spent time during the workday getting cards signed.

Ultimately, the NYSNA won the election with 53 percent of the vote to the trade unions' 43 percent. The League of Registered Nurses, Local 1199, won only 9 percent of the vote; the Federation of Nurses/UFT won 34 percent; and 4 percent of the votes were challenged.

Nursing Unionism at St. John's Hospital

Registered nurses at St. John's Hospital had been members of the League of Registered Nurses Local 1199 since 1980, having encountered problems similar to those endured by Mt. Zion nurses. Aides and LPNs were being laid off after years of loyal service to the hospital, and registered nurses who remained were expected to carry the workload themselves. On top of a deteriorating staff-patient ratio, the RNs lacked control over such work conditions as health and safety, indiscriminate promotions, merit raises, suspensions, and incidents of racial discrimination. During their tenure with Local 1199, these conditions began to change. Management began to comply with grievance procedures and follow through on salary and promotion schedules mutually agreed upon with the union. Nurses began to feel more in control at work. Then the leadership at the top of

Local 1199 changed, turning their world upside down.

Until 1982, Local 1199 had been known as "the union with soul," a strong supporter of civil rights and peace during the Vietnam era. It was composed primarily of African-American and female unskilled workers until the mid-1970s, at which time it had launched a major drive to organize technical, clerical, and nursing workers. These workers were organized into separate Guild and Nursing Divisions, the latter of which was officially organized by Sondra Clarke in 1977.

By this time, Local 1199 had expanded its list of health benefits; had a credit union, academic scholarships, and summer camp stipends for workers' children; and supported such issues as community-controlled schools, rent strikes, and a cultural program entitled, Bread and Roses, which brought live theater to thousands of union members during their lunch hours (Fink, 1986: 183-84). It was known as Martin Luther King's favorite union.

In 1982, all this came to a halt. Doris Turner, a former dietary aide, was the hand-picked successor by Leon Davis, who had been in the leadership for five decades. As a religious black woman, Turner rejected Davis's cultural and political values in favor of greater reliance on religious prayer. She negated the unity Davis had fostered among the different divisions in the union and rejected his focus on interracialism and peace policies. She drove a wedge between herself and the existing leadership as well as the membership. Twelve of 14 guild organizers and 12 district vice presidents were forced out (Fink, 1986; Klein, 1985), including a former head of the nursing division who claimed "Turner wasn't the least bit interested in nurses" (S. Clarke, former head of RN Division, 1985). The membership, now comprising of both uneducated, unskilled minority women and educated, skilled technical men and women, was also becoming rigidly divided. Turner's priority was decidedly with the former group (which did not include nurses).

Nurses from St. John's Hospital described their personal experiences with Turner at the delegates' assembly. They felt ostracized and abused by her. She uttered nasty comments toward them in public, issuing commands to "shut up and sit down" at delegate meetings. She derided them for appearing "too good to be associated with everyone else." Nurses were being driven away by Turner, and they stopped going to the delegates' assembly meetings.

The culmination of Turner's divisive management style was her defiant negotiating stance taken with hospitals in 1984. Despite the fact that New York State was reducing reimbursement rates to hospitals, Local 1199 demanded a 5 percent salary increase and every other weekend off (a benefit 80 percent of the membership already had), rejecting the hospital's compromise of 26 weekends off and a 4 percent pay raise. Turner called for an unprecedented six-week city-wide strike, although she had not discussed this prospect with her executive committee. One of her former executive vice presidents, David White (from the Guild Division), was so distraught with what Turner was doing to the union that he went public with her actions in November 1984 to the Department of Labor and in

1985 to the press ("Turnergate" audiotape, David White interviewed by Dennis Rivera: current 1199 president, 1984). White claimed that Turner was holding the strike simply to make political hay and outdo Leon Davis, who was known for a 46-day strike. Nurses started leaving the union in droves.

The nurses' contract at St. John's was not up until October 1984. From the start, their participation in the strike was in sympathy with the Hospital and Guild divisions. Two hundred nurses finally went out on strike from St. John's, although no union officers or representatives accompanied them on their picket lines. They were also unable to get any information about the progress of negotiations, and instructions about their own participation were nil.

Neither St. John's nor the three other hospitals where nurses were striking had received the required 10-day filing notice of a sympathy strike (resulting in exorbitant fines for Local 1199), although the union had told the nurses this matter was already taken care of (Fink and Greenberg, 1989: 224). St. John's took advantage of this disarray. It intimidated nurses one-on-one, holding them in management offices until late into the night, and telling them that a court order was out for them. Management harassed them with intimidating phone calls at home, and at St. Barnabus Hospital, where nurses were also striking, the hot water was turned off in the nurses' residence hall for the duration of the strike (*Unity and Progress News*, 1984: 10). The hospital took advantage of nurses' general feeling of betrayal by Local 1199 and knew the union had become a paper tiger.

The striking nurses became so frustrated that at 3 a.m. one morning, after almost two weeks of walking the picket line, they went to Roosevelt Hotel, where Local 1199's leadership was staying for the duration, to find out what was going on. They were refused entrance by Turner henchmen, and were told that if they did not leave the premises, the police would be sent out to arrest them. Former executive vice-president David White finally exposed the bacchanalian activities of Turner and her staff during this period. They had rented lavish hotel rooms at $500 a night and were occupying themselves with continual card games, champagne and expensive food (White, 1984, "Turnergate Tapes").

The last straw was when Turner tampered with the Local 1199 elections, held in May 1984. She was up against a powerful Slate 2 opposition, known as the Unity and Progress Group, and she was discarding ballots (primarily from the Nursing and Guild divisions) marked in favor of her opponents. By April 1986, the Department of Labor supervised another election, and Slate 2 won, placing Georgianna Johnson, an African-American, 55-year-old former social work assistant, in Turner's position as president. By this time, nurses in four different hospitals had decertified Local 1199 in favor of NYSNA, the organization that many at St. John's saw as their only alternative.

Nurses at St. John's were caught in the wake of general corruption that had permeated Local 1199's leadership between 1982 and 1986. During Sondra Clarke's tenure as the head of the Nurses' Division, St. John's nurses had developed a real trust in the union and a belief in its ideals. Clarke resigned in

1983 due to her conflict with the Turner leadership. The nurses felt their relationship with the union had begun crumbling since that point. The atmosphere for nurses at both St. John's and Mt. Zion hospitals was clearly emotionally charged regarding issues of unionism.[12]

OVERVIEW

Chapter 2 provides an in-depth analysis of some of the issues mentioned in this introduction: the transformation of the organization of work in the United States since 1870, the rise of white collar workers, and concomitant changes in the nursing occupation. It examines the emergence of professionalism in nursing and other, more independent professions. Finally, it examines the ways in which the three different collective strategies emerge in nursing.

Chapter 3 analyzes in detail nurses' class position, using Wright's framework. It examines each nursing segment's level of control within the economic, political, and ideological realms of production.

Chapter 4 demonstrates the way in which nurses' class position has a determining effect on their class identity (indicated by their choice of collective strategy), mediated by their interpretations of professionalism. That is, it examines in detail the emergence of different interpretations of professionalism (work control; capitalist individualism; and a composite of the two, work control and popular individualism) in relation to class position and collective actions.

Finally, the conclusion to this study suggests that salaried, educated, white collar workers comprise different contradictory class locations. This group is made up of distinct segments, crosscutting occupations, with different levels of control in the labor process. Their subjective class identity and forms of collective action reflect this objective heterogeneity. Workers in each class position convey their own maps of social reality, their own ideologies, around which they collectively organize. Thus, some identify with the values and strategies of organized labor, some with the values and strategies of individualized forms of social mobility, and some with certain values and strategies of both organized labor and individual mobility.

This study empirically demonstrates that the fastest-growing sector of the American labor force, the educated white collar work force, is objectively stratified, displaying no evidence of unified class politics.

NOTES

1. Managed competition theoretically means that individuals will be clustered into large, state-organized purchasing groups, or health alliances. Ostensibly, a wide range of health providers would rise up and compete for the sponsor's business. In addition, a

variety of federal subsidies (to poor people and small employers), and regulations to limit deductibles, would set minimum benefit packages and encourage all the actors (employers, employees, sponsors, states, health plans, and individual providers), to act in socially responsible ways (Morone, 1992; Starr, 1993).

2.   In the past two decades this trend has picked up considerable momentum due to deindustrialization, the loss of blue collar manufacturing work in the United States, and the rise of low-wage, nonunion, white collar service sector work (Bluestone and Harrison, 1982, 1988; Kuttner, 1984; Reich, 1992).

3.   According to the 19990 U.S. Census, between 1977 and 1989, three-fourths of the gain in pretax income went to the wealthiest 660,000 families, a 77 percent gain. At the same time, the family in the middle income range rose only 4 percent, to $36,000 (Newman, 1993).

4.   They instituted a no-strike policy in 1950, which was lifted in 1964 due to pressure placed upon them by the membership as members began choosing trade unions over the professional union. Nevertheless, the NYSNA employs a Nurses in Dispute Policy, which states that "nurses should maintain a scrupulously neutral position in regard to labor management relations between their employers and non-nurses employees." Thus, solidarity with other hospital workers is still forbidden by NYSNA.

5.   Control over the labor process is implied in the discussion of Edwards's notion of control within the firm. Edwards illustrates in detail that control is of such import to owners that they would rather pay high wages than relinquish control over work pace, length of day, or knowledge of the process of production. Similarly, control is important to all nurses in this study, whether it is over particular tasks or the occupation as a whole. Hence, I endorse Wright's focus on control relations.

6.   See Table 1.1 for a summary of this study's findings on the relationship of nurses' class position, choice of strategy, and interpretation of professionalism.

7.   The survey was coded according to the following variables: Class Location, Collective Strategy, Symbol of Professionalism, Class Identity, Work History, and Demographic Data. (See Appendix B.) The hypotheses were evaluated by a count of all the cases. For nurses in each class position, I examined the number who chose a particular collective strategy, why they said they chose it, and their understanding of professionalism. (See Table 1.1.)

8.   I had sent in formal applications to nursing directors at three different hospitals (at their request) and was rejected each time. Although I never received a reason for their rejection of my proposal, I concluded, after having completed this study, that the nursing administrators reviewing my questionnaire (with several questions on unionism) did not want a researcher to stir up their staff with questions on collective organization. Issues about unionism are very alive and threatening to cost-conscious hospital administrators.

Other forms of data, such as change over time in types of nonmedical workers, proved similarly difficult to obtain

9.   Fantasia criticizes the use of traditional sociological survey instruments for similar reasons, particularly in studies of class consciousness. He argues that surveys tend to record only fixed, static responses, not the subtleties and contradictions inherent in the development of class consciousness and the building of solidarity (Fantasia, 1988: ch. 1).

10.   In addition, the Rns worked closely with physicians and were exposed to the doctors' more individualist, human capital interpretation of professionalism: pursuit of credentialism to attain social and economic status.

11. NYSNA, however, had told the nurses it did not agree to an arbitrator to settle the dispute.

12. The rampant corruption and disarray of Local 1199 during the period of this research might raise questions about the validity of nurses' reactions to trade unionism, given the exceptionalism of the union in question. This potential confusion was clarified, however, by nurses' class-linked interpretations of professionalism. That is, while 60 percent of the nurses in a low class position supported trade unionism as a collective strategy, 84 percent defined professionalism as work control: control over the conditions of work, the thrust of trade unionism.

Chapter 2

Rise of the White Collar Worker, Ideology of Professionalism, and White Collar Strategies: The Case of Nursing

A variety of economic and political processes transformed the organization of work beginning in the 1870s. These transformations gave rise to new occupations, changing a vast component of the American workforce into what are known collectively as white collar workers, though some enjoy nearly complete control over their work while others are virtually unable to exercise any discretion on the job at all. Along with the emergence of white collar work came a human capital interpretation of professionalism--a stalwart belief in individualized means of attaining social and economic status. According to this ideology, such status is achieved through increased educational credentialism and "proper behaviors." As these new salaried, white collar workers fought to secure some degree of autonomy in the workplace, they legitimized their struggle with the human capital ideology.

The occupation of nursing was, like other white collar pursuits, subject to pressures of diminished control and became enmeshed in struggles among different interpretations of professionalism. There are, indeed, very different segments within the nursing workforce, which, according to position in the workplace, have regarded very differently the ideology of professionalism. In addition, each group within nursing has employed a different organizational strategy to secure its goals: professionalization, professional unionism, or trade unionization. In each case, ownership over the imagery of the professional, as either educated expert or experienced, autonomous worker, became the focal point in the battle for workplace control.

TRANSFORMATION OF WORK

It is critical to situate nursing within a broader context of economic and occupational change in order to understand its stratified workforce and divergent responses to the work environment. Between 1870 and 1920, the organization of work in the United States underwent a major transformation. Monopoly capitalism superseded competitive capitalism, and huge firms with large workforces were formed. The small, independent entrepreneur was dwarfed by comparison.

During the 1870s, the American business cycle experienced contraction, and economic instability ensued. Firms began to protect themselves from the threat of bankruptcy and competition by forming trusts and monopolies. This movement of mergers and consolidations increased the power and profits of such industries as steel, oil, and the railroads, resulting in the demise of small merchants and manufacturers (Edwards, 1979; Wiebe, 1967; Gordon, Edwards, and Reich, 1982; Lipow, 1982). The massive wealth and power of this newly emerging group of millionaires dwarfed the power and prestige of the old petite bourgeoisie. Hofstadter writes, "The newly rich, the grandiosely or corruptly rich, the masters of the great corporation were bypassing . . . the old gentry, the merchants of longstanding, the small manufacturers, the established professional men and the civic leaders of an earlier era" (Hofstadter, 1955: 137).

As prospects in business and farming deteriorated for the self-employed, two new forms of white collar employment presented themselves: (1) salaried employment within the new corporate firm and (2) self-employment within one of the old professions, such as medicine, law, or dentistry.

Salaried Employment within the Firm

Salaried employment within the firm was the option most readily available for the majority of men.[1] As ownership became separated from management and as the size of the new firm increased, opportunities for employment emerged at the managerial level, fulfilling the need to control a larger workforce.

Principles of scientific management put forth by Frederick Taylor were beginning to appear in the 1870s, calling for the separation between hand and brain in production. Management was to become the brain and workers the hands (Taylor, 1947). Management appropriated the knowledge of production from workers and divided their tasks into component parts. Such a system, which deprived the skilled worker of his craft secrets and skills, created a much greater role for various levels of management (Montgomery, 1979).

A managerial workforce was henceforth required to plan, design, and supervise the production processes. Thus, an entirely new stratum of workers emerged: engineers to design the technical aspects of production and supervisors to manage the social aspects of production (Edwards, 1979; Noble, 1977).

Braverman's eloquent description of this separation between hand and brain in the new corporate labor process deserves to be repeated:

Separate sites and separate bodies of workers. In one location, the physical processes of production [were] executed. In another . . . the design, planning, calculation and record keeping [were concentrated]. . . . The production units operated like a hand; watched, connected and controlled, by a distant brain. (Braverman, 1974: 124-5)

Not only were engineers and supervisors needed for the new corporate firm, but so were a variety of salesmen, market forecasters, and advertisers as well. As production increased, workers were needed to measure the market demand for particular products, sell them, and create a demand for that product within the potential market. Entire white collar industries in advertising, insurance, banking, and finance developed in response (Edwards, 1979). Thus, whereas in 1820, 72 percent of the labor force was in farming, by 1870, that number had decreased to 53 percent, and, by 1900, it had fallen to 37 percent. By 1900, 18 percent of the total workforce were managers, supervisors, salesmen, and other types of high-level, salaried, white collar workers (U.S. Department of Commerce, Bureau of Census, 1976).

Alongside the rise of high-level salaried employment came an increasing demand for low-level, salaried employees in clerical and service work. Women, seeking to avoid the drudgery of factory labor in the mills of New England, found opportunities available in these two forms of cleaner, albeit degraded, employment (Davies, 1982; Reverby, 1987). As more desirable white collar occupations opened up within the bureaucratically controlled organization, men were hired, leaving the low-level white collar work (mainly clerical and service work) to women (Stroeber, 1984; Stroeber and Arnold, 1987). This work often resembled production work in that both were subject to similar processes of de-skilling (Davies, 1982; Glenn and Feldberg, 1981; Ehrenreich and Ehrenreich, 1971, 1976). Clerical work, for example, was divided into its component parts, such as filing, billing, typing, and stenography. Once a stepping-stone to management for some males within the small firm, feminized clerical work lost all forms of job mobility and became a low-paid occupation (Davies, 1982).

Service work followed similar lines of development. As small communities and extended families were torn asunder by wage labor with the rise of monopoly capitalism, large institutions began to replace family functions of caring for the sick, the old, and the indigent (Ryan, 1984; Braverman, 1974). Family members left the household for wage work and were no longer able to care for their own (Epstein, 1982). Thus, large-scale employment of service workers emerged in such institutions as schools, hospitals, and prisons. This work was performed primarily by women who were, like female clerical workers, low paid, with minimal job mobility, and minimal control over their labor process (Ehrenreich and Ehrenreich, 1971; Reverby, 1987; Kessler-Harris, 1986; Stroeber and Arnold, 1987).

Two seemingly distinct trends were therefore intimately intertwined: (1) the decrease in independent entrepreneurs and farmers and (2) the rise of two distinct types of salaried, white collar employees within the corporate firm: those with greater levels of control over their work processes (managers, engineers, and salesmen) and those with minimal levels of control over their work processes (clerical and service workers) (Oppenheimer, 1985).

The Role of Education

Education was part and parcel of this transformation in occupational structure. As early as the 1890s, corporate financiers were devising ways to control the direction of education to meet their own needs. On the one hand they wanted a more disciplined, compliant, productive workforce. On the other, they wanted a subservient managerial and supervisory workforce, subordinate to the needs of the corporation.

In 1890, J. P. Morgan and John D. Rockefeller provided major financial backing for the development of vocational education, while other tycoons supported the growth of the new university (Brint and Karabel, 1989; Bowles and Gintis, 1976; Vesey, 1965; Larson, 1979). Between 1890 and 1910, business leaders became the predominant group on university boards of trustees.

These corporate leaders had specific business goals for the new educational enterprise. Support for expanded public education was predicated on the notion that education for the masses would diminish resistance both within and outside the workplace. Public school would discipline, train, and "Americanize" the working class, many of whom were immigrants, and between 1890 and 1930, the public high school became a mass institution. In 1890 only 4 percent of the 17-year-old population had graduated from high school. By 1930, this figure rose to 29 percent (Bowles and Gintis, 1976).

Labor was well aware of the hidden agenda undergirding the public educational system, as a statement by the Chicago Federation of Labor indicates:

[Such a system] reflects an effort on the part of large employers to turn the public schools into an agency for supplying them with an adequate supply of docile, well trained, and capable workers . . . aimed to bring Illinois a caste system of education which would shunt the children of the laboring classes at an early age first into vocational education and then into the factories. (quoted in Karabel, 1972: 550)

While public education was supported by big business for the purpose of "taming" the working class, the new university was supported in order to harness scientific innovation and managerial techniques to the corporation. Leland Stanford, for example, a railroad tycoon, funnelled millions of dollars into Stanford University to create a school of engineering. He appointed David Starr Jordan, a businessman, as president of the university. Jordan fought for the pragmatic needs of business to dominate the school's curriculum, arguing that "reality and practicality," not esoteric theory, should be the raison d'etre of the new university movement (Vesey, 1965). Similarly, Andrew Draper, president of the

University of Illinois, argued that "higher education should prepare students for all skilled employments . . . in the constructive and commercial industries" (Vesey, 1965: 71).

It is within this business-oriented context, then, that salaried, white collar workers such as engineers were socialized to remain subordinate to the needs of the corporation. In speaking to a graduating class of engineers in 1896, the president of an engineering alumni group, the Stevens Institute Alumni Association, stated, "The sooner the young engineer recedes from the idea that simply because he is a `professional man,' his position is paramount, the better for him. . . . He must always be subservient to those who represent the money invested in the enterprise" (Noble, 1979: 35).

Thus, engineers, once independent, skilled craftsmen, were transformed into educated, salaried employees, subordinate to the needs of the corporation (Noble, 1977; Larson, 1977; Zussman, 1985). Clearly business leaders of the late 19th and early 20th centuries attempted to mold the educational system in accord with their own needs, contributing to the transformation of the occupational system.[2]

Movements toward Professionalization

Many members of the old petite bourgeoisie at the end of the 19th century partook in this education movement in order to avert their own demise, and they sought opportunity in the various professions. Rather than become salaried employees, subordinate to the dictates of the new corporate world, they sought economic independence in the fields of medicine, law, and dentistry. Between 1870 and 1890 these professions more than doubled in size (Lipow, 1982: 142).

During that period, the professions were hardly what they are today. Robert Wiebe describes the professional of the 1880s as basically any individual who chose to hang up a shingle:

The concept of a middle class crumbled at the touch. Small businesses appeared and disappeared at a frightening rate. The so called professions meant little as long as anyone with a bag of pills and bottle of syrup could pass for a doctor, a few books and a corrupt judge made a man a lawyer, and an unemployed literate qualified as a "teacher."
What they all shared was nothing more than a common sense of drift . . . a salary, a set of clean clothes and hope that somehow they would rise in the world. (Wiebe, 1967: 13-14)

In self-defense against the corporate consolidations, members of the "old American gentry" (as Hofstadter refers to them)--the farmers, small capitalists, and intellectuals--banded together to seek their own solution. They turned toward the state for protection of their interests, demanding legislation to "avert the doom of small property." As Lewis Corey put it:

The state was to regulate the freedom of enterprise and competition; to limit the rights of property in the interests of small property. This was a formidable shift on the part of middle class radicals [who had previously supported laissez-faire]. They now urged limitation of the economic freedom which they formerly believed was sufficient in itself to realize the economic equality of a society of small producers. Where formerly they demanded abolition of all political privileges, they now wanted them restored in the interest of the small enterpriser. (Corey, 1935: 129-30)

Members of this reform coalition solicited state sponsorship for control over occupational markets. Through the device of licensing, they drew the state into the task of credentialing the professions, thus preventing those unlicensed from practicing. The members of the old American gentry involved in this movement for professionalization attempted to transform special skills and knowledge, expertise, into economic and social rewards. Such a task, according to Larson, could be accomplished only by gaining state-sponsored monopoly control over that expertise (Larson, 1977).

This was achieved in the late 19th century by creating state-accredited educational programs within the new universities. Each profession carved out academic disciplines that secured its claims to special expertise. With the development of accredited programs, in schools such as engineering, medicine, law, business administration, and nursing, only those professionals who had been officially licensed would be allowed to practice, thereby eliminating competition from the unlicensed. Through this mechanism, professionals running educational programs were able to act as gatekeepers, controlling their schools. By reducing the number of practitioners at the point of entry, a scarcity of expertise could be created within an occupation, enhancing the economic reward for practicing professionals (Larson, 1977; Collins, 1979: ch. 6). The result was a near-monopoly control over the market for professional services.

Yet not all occupations were successful in implementing this strategy of professionalization. According to Larson (1977), only occupations that could control the point of entry and exchange their services directly with clients were able to achieve true monopoly control. Most other professional occupations were unable to get this far. Fields like nursing, engineering, social work, and school administration were dependent on business or the state for their market and did not exchange their services directly with clients. This prevented them from achieving full control over their own economic situations. Although they may have controlled the point of entry (the numbers entering the occupation through the professional schools), they remained dependent, salaried employees, unable to control the larger market forces affecting their employment. If, for example, the business climate was favorable, engineers might be hired by businesses. If that climate was unfavorable, they might find themselves unemployed. Unable to control fluctuations in the business cycle, such salaried employees were unable to control the market for their services.

In contrast, doctors and lawyers exchanged their service with clients without any mediating institutions (e.g., the state). They could therefore control not only the entry point into their occupation (and, hence, the numbers of practitioners, by guarding the gates to their professional schools) but were able to determine the fees and conditions for the services they provided as well. These independent professional entrepreneurs were in a better position to exert monopoly control over their own market.

Dependent, salaried professionals (such as hospital nurses), unable to reap economic rewards because of their very dependence as an occupation, were able to achieve social status from professionalization. Larson maintains that boosting prestige through an affiliation with higher education and professional occupations was important to that middle strata in late-19th-century America, as they were being socially and financially marginalized by the rising corporate structures, diminishing possibilities for independent practitioners (Larson, 1977). The professionalization effort was thus suffused with an ideology of elitism, embodied within the construct of professionalism. Those affiliated with higher learning, pursuing educational credentials, who aspired to serve the public good, considered themselves above the working class. To become a professional was therefore to boost one's social position.

This individualized means of self-improvement, reflected in the human capital construct of professionalism, provided salaried professionals with a sense of self-esteem. It was, nevertheless, a double-edged sword, for simultaneously it served as a system of control in the workplace. Professionalism imparted a sense of status to the salaried professional worker, yet it also provided employers with an invisible form of control over employees (Stone, 1975; Edwards, 1979). Firms were able to provide the illusion of job mobility as employers instituted artificial job ladders. They created rungs on the professional occupational ladder with increased status but little variation in autonomy or pay. These artificial job ladders enabled employers to provide professional workers with a sense of promotion, while maintaining their subordination to higher levels of managerial authority.

Nursing exemplifies such a professional occupational ladder, with countless rungs leading up, but not high up. In ascending order, registered nurses can become staff nurse, senior clinical nurse, clinical supervisor, division coordinator, assistant director, associate director, and vice president for nursing. Although the top three levels are more administrative, with higher salaries than the others, all nursing levels are subordinate to an array of physicians and hospital administrators. These nurses are all perceived by their superiors as ultimately interchangeable, regardless of the fact that the later categories perform adminis-trative, not clinical, duties.

Unionization was prevented or forestalled by the human capital, individualist notion of professionalism as well. Professionals were reluctant to align them-selves with labor unions, the classic symbol of the working class. Instead, professionals were more likely to form professional organizations, attend professional meetings, and write for professional journals rather than join trade unions. This in turn dampened the spread of the union movement since the burgeoning white collar professions sought to protect status gains by forming associations within the workplace to represent their aspirations.

Finally, the individualist vision of professionalism serves to encourage Individual as opposed to Collective advancement in the workplace in terms of salary increases, benefits, and work conditions. That is, individual social mobility was promoted, to be attained through such personal means as educational credentialism and the display of proper behavior.

Collective advancement pursued through such processes as collective bargaining, intrinsic to trade unionism, was again portrayed as nonprofessional, since it pit worker against employer. According to the individualist vision of professionalism, such a contest in the workplace would be unnecessary if proper behaviors were employed. Individuals would rationally work out their problems with their employer. Individual advancement that pits worker against worker thus deflects blame from management and places it more squarely on the individual. With laser-beam acuity, the weaknesses of the individual, rather than the structural problems of the workplace, are highlighted. Thus, the individualist interpretation of professionalism became a powerful, invisible, cultural message enabling employers to gain a more compliant, self-controlled workforce (Larson, 1979; Edwards, 1979; Stone, 1975).

This vision of professionalism draws on the culture of meritocracy, a dominant thread throughout American cultural history, derived from the Protestant ethic (Newman, 1988). Katherine Newman suggests that high-level white collar workers such as corporate executives perceive their rise and fall in occupational and social status as a result of their own inherent abilities. Such a Social Darwinist view negates the influences of external factors' determining one's place in society, such as fluctuations in the overall economy or unequal opportunity structures, and once again serves to pit workers against themselves and each other.

NURSING: A CONFLICT BETWEEN CLASSES AND COLLECTIVE STRATEGIES

The history of nursing, a segment of the white collar service sector, reflects the general trends in the transformation of work that gave rise to the new, dependent, salaried, white collar workforce, in conflict over the construct of professionalism. Although previously independent practitioners, by the end of World War II, a decisive majority of nurses were forced to find employment in the newly emerging bureaucratic hospitals as their opportunities for autonomous nurse-patient relationships diminished (Melosh, 1982). In the nation's hospitals, nurses were subject to processes of bureaucratic control very much like those described by Edwards for both production and nonproduction workers (Edwards, 1979).

Invisible mechanisms of control, including the human capital notion of professionalism and the use of written rules to govern nurses' tasks and supervision, were invoked to discipline this white collar workforce.

Historically, nurses' responses to these constraints have been filled with conflict. On the one hand, some have attempted to professionalize, particularly nurses who had experienced a decline in their middle-class status. Nurses from the working class, on the other hand, attempted to organize into trade unions. Finally, we find attempts at professional unionization by nurses from both the working and middle classes who occupied middle managerial positions. In order to understand these divergent trends we must look at a more detailed history of the nursing profession.

Working-Class Origins of Nursing

In the 18th century, nursing was merely another of womens' domestic chores.[3] By the early 19th century, however, nursing had emerged as an occupation performed by respectable working-class women, primarily widows and spinsters. It was a specialty within domestic service, consisting primarily of cleaning a patient's body, linen, and dressings. This kind of labor was considered by most 19th-century men and women as an extension of woman's "natural" biological capacity for domesticity, docility, nurturance, and willingness to sacrifice (Berg, 1978).

A fine line separated the 19th-century nurse from the domestic servant, as both were expected to perform household chores. By 1868, however, they were more clearly differentiated by salary; the nurse earned $1.00 to $2.00 a day whereas the servant earned only $2.22 per week (Reverby, 1987). Because of the close association with dirty domestic work, few middle-class women entered nursing. Until the Civil War, nursing remained an occupation performed by poor, older, single women with no formal education or training. These women were often drawn from rural areas into the cities in search of paid work, where their options were generally sewing, lodging borders, domestic service, or nursing.[4] By 1870, there were over 10,000 women officially employed as nurses in the United States.

Until the 20th century, hospital nursing was less prevalent than household nursing since most births, deaths, and illnesses occurred in the home (Vogel, 1980). The majority of Americans did not see the inside of a hospital until the turn of the century. Hospitals were barely hospitals as we now know them. They were charitable institutions built by philanthropists at the end of the 18th century for the poor, the socially marginal, or the unemployed. Indeed, many hospitals evolved out of public almshouses. Patients in both public and voluntary hospitals were incarcerated for dependence as much as for disease in the 1870s (Vogel, 1980: 105), and their hospital stay was often for weeks or months, not days. Impermeable walls and guarded gates surrounded the institutions, enabling hospitals to assert some control over the working class, immigrant, or destitute patient.

Although benevolent, hospitals treated their patients disdainfully, with authoritarianism and paternalism. Their purpose was to provide the patient with moral uplift while instilling social control. Hospital administrators believed their patients were from "the very lowest; from abodes of drunkenness and vice in almost every form, where the most depressing and corrupting influences were acting on both body and mind" (Vogel, 1980: 24). Children were decontaminated upon arrival and taught "discipline, purity and kindness." The trustees hoped this regimen would reform the children, who would then bring "newly refined manners, quickened intellect and softened hearts" back to their homes. Some hospitals attempted to reform adults as well because they believed society benefited not just by saving these workers but also by "rekindling in them their faith in social order" (Vogel, 1980: 26).

Nurses in these hospitals were generally ambulatory patients themselves, caring for fellow "inmates." If not actual patients, hospital nurses originated from the same poor and working-class sectors of society as the patients. They often held several jobs simultaneously and were frequently reprimanded for "sewing-out" (manufacturing garments on the ward) while on duty (Reverby, 1987).

The status of the 19th-century hospital nurse was very low, comparable to the status of all female patients at this time. The female patient of 1870 was characterized in a letter to the *Boston Evening Transcript* as "a woman who has fallen into the sins of the wayside . . . too weak to resist the temptations which have beset their unguarded footsteps" (Vogel, 1980: 26). Similarly, the hospital nurse was characterized by Florence Nightingale, the 19th-century British reformer, as "too old, too weak, too drunk, too dirty, too stolid or too bad to do anything else" (quoted in Reverby, 1987: 26). Hence, stringent rules governing general behaviors regarding sex, language, and use of alcohol and tobacco were enforced for both patients and nurses in the hospital.

Although nurses lived in close proximity to the patients, they were forbidden to socialize with them. In order to prevent them from socializing or drinking with the patients, nurses were kept busy from 5:00 a.m. until 9:30 p.m. They were continually scrubbing patients, garments, and wards, since sanitation was the only method of disease prevention in the 19th-century hospital. When they had completed these tasks, they were given innumerable others to keep them in line.

In addition to such domestic tasks, nurses were often responsible for providing more serious health care in the doctor's frequent absence as well. They often managed labor and delivery cases independently. This forced nurses to exercise independent medical judgments, despite doctors' prevailing expectation that nurses would be completely subservient to them. With the taste of autonomy, nurses began to expect greater latitude in their work. They began to see themselves as adult wage workers, not children to be controlled by the hospital "family," as the hospital trustees portrayed the workplace.

Middle-Class Women Attempt Transformation of Nursing

The face of nursing changed during the Civil War. Middle- and upper-class women, motivated by patriotism, familial duty, or simply a search for meaningful work, began to work in hospitals, nursing wounded men, and raising funds for the war (Mottus, 1980: 65). The unsanitary and disorganized conditions in army hospitals led to the emergence of relief associations. In 1861 the Women's Central Association of Relief was formed with the explicit purpose of "furnishing comforts and medical stores, and especially nurses in aid of the medical staff of the army . . . and to take measures for securing a system of well trained nurses against any possible demand of war" (Mottus, 1980: 24). Drawing on Nightingale's British model of army nursing, the Registration Committee on Nurses sought prospective applicants with specific qualifications: they were to wear dresses without hoops, provide references confirming their high moral character, and be no older than 45 years of age. Nurses trained according to Nightingale's nursing model, learning the laws of both morality and hygiene.

The post-Civil War years, characterized by remarkable economic growth, the rise of industrial corporations, the decline of small entrepreneurs, and the emergence of urban America, engendered the expansion of relief organizations and the development of new charity organizations. Both were controlled in large part by middle- and upper-class female reformers. These women, many of whom had participated in organized nursing during the Civil War, focused on reforming the moral character of the poor, soiled by the ravages of urban society (Kessler-Harris, 1982; Lubove, 1965). The expansion of the charity organization movement represented another response by a troubled middle class to the social dislocation of the post-Civil War industrial city: "Charity organization was a crusade to save the city from itself and from the evils of pauperism and class antagonism. It was an instrument of social control for the conservative middle class" (Lubove, 1965: 5).[5]

In the post-Civil War hospital, middle-class women joined forces with hospital trustees and developed training schools for nurses. The reformers' purpose was to "save" the country girl from the city, foster a profession of nursing, and reform the hospital. They attempted to carry out this goal by developing a cadre of trained, professional, middle-class nurses. The hospital trustees, however, sought nurses as a cheap labor force for the hospital.

During the depression years of the 1890s, the hospital moved away from being a charity organization (Rosner, 1986: 119). Philanthropists, affected by financial crises themselves, were no longer able to be the sole supporters of the institutions. Hospital trustees turned to the middle-class patient as a new source of income for hospitals. This change motivated trustees to alter the hospital's architecture as well as its workforce. Its image became more hotel-like, with private rooms, private doctors, and private nurses. The reformers convinced the trustees that young, educated nurses of middle-class origins would be more appropriate caretakers for wealthier patients than untrained, working-class nurses (Mottus, 1980). Hence, while the middle-class reformers were attempting to create a profession for respectable middle-class women, embodying Victorian America's idealized vision of upper-class womanhood (empathy, gentility, and dedication to service), the trustees were still seeking an inexpensive yet disciplined workforce. The middle-class student nurse was their answer.

One of the first training schools for nurses emerged in 1889 at the Johns Hopkins Hospital as a joint effort between the women reformers and the hospital trustees. They sought applications from Episcopalian and Presbyterian daughters of the clergy and the professions (James, 1979: 214). The reformers hoped such a school would become the new social incubator for daughters of the new middle class. They sought only educated and refined students; women who had previously worked in the mills or domestic service were discouraged from applying. The reformers argued that only women with proper, virtuous backgrounds could enhance the moral atmosphere of the hospital.

Blue Collar Character of Nursing Remains with the Occupation

In reality, nursing school was not simply a breeding ground for daughters of the middle class. Because the schools were financially dependent on the hospital and its needs for cheap labor, most were forced to admit women with less education from working-class backgrounds in order to meet the hospital's needs.[6] Admission to nursing school was thus determined by the hospital's labor requirements, not the educator's desired admission standards.

Student nurses worked in the hospital; their training was secondary. In fact, their work closely resembled that of their untrained counterparts, and physicians often called them "hospital machines." As one student nurse stated in the 1870s, quoted by Sara Parsons in her history of the Massachusetts General Hospital Training School:

We did the sweeping in all the wards and ward corridors. . . . We washed the bedsteads and bedside tables. If the head nurse was very particular about the looks of her ward we had to mop it every day.... We did the dusting, we carried the clothes to the laundry and the poultice clothes and used bandages to the rinse house. . . . We washed dishes twice a day, for we had but one maid for three wards. (quoted in Reverby, 1987:106)

Student nurse training meant working 13-hour days at domestic duties under strict military discipline. Understaffing and medical emergency continually forced students into positions for which they were unprepared. These poor work conditions of overwork, lack of adequate training, bad food, and arbitrary discipline took their toll on the students, resulting in the 1910s in strikes against nursing supervisors (Reverby, 1987).

The Problem of "Unprofessional Behavior"

Nursing superintendents, who were generally educated women of middle-class origin, warned their staff against these strikes, as they were reminiscent of working-class behavior. These educators and supervisors were desperately trying to escape from this lower status image, as this 1915 report from *Trained Nurse* indicates:

> Any nurse is justified in showing her disapproval of conditions or actions by resigning in a dignified way, and, sometimes, doing it on short notice. But the methods of this "sympathy strike" savor so strongly of labor unions that those who have retained the old fashioned ideals of nursing taught by Florence Nightingale can hardly help gasping and exclaiming, "what next!" (quoted in Reverby, 1987: 119)

Nursing students of both working- and middle-class origins were bombarded by the human capital ethos of professionalism. Dedication to service, gentility, and rejection of all working-class behavior were prerequisites for the job. This ideological onslaught left many students conflicted over the legitimacy of strike tactics.

Nursing educators and supervisors suffered no such confusion, they aimed squarely at the professionalization of nursing. By the 1890s they had begun their attempts to enhance the occupation's, as well as their own, personal, economic, and social status, limiting the occupation to the middle class (Mottus, 1980; James, 1979). Two major nursing associations were established as the force behind this movement of professionalization: the American Society of Superintendents of Training Schools in the United States and Canada, later to become the National League of Nursing Education (NLNE), and the Nurse's Associated Alumnae of the United States and Canada, later to become the ANA.

These associations sought to establish standards of entry that once again emphasized proper middle-class character. This was soon transformed into "proper educational background," which became a mechanism for excluding working-class women from the occupation. Education was a measurable proxy for class background, since, as one superintendent wrote in *Trained Nurse and Hospital Review* in 1897, "It's easier to maintain a criterion from an educational standpoint than from a moral or social aspect" (quoted in Reverby, 1982: 224).

Intense appeals to the middle-class effectively alienated the majority of working-class nurses from the professionalizers. Staff nurses of working-class origins began to speak out on their need to work and their desire for improved work conditions. They rejected the human capital interpretation of professionalism, clearly illustrated in this 1888 letter to *Trained Nurse*, by none other than "Candor":

> Where there is one nurse with a missionary spirit . . . there are forty-nine others who are obliged to make the humiliating confession: I am a nurse because I must earn a living for

myself and those dependent on me, because my nursing is well-paid, honorable, and to me interesting. . . . Of course this spirit of self immolation is very beautiful and lovely, but is it practical?

Let us be honest, even at the sacrifice of sentiment. Let us not hesitate to do a good deed when opportunity offers, but let us not try to make people believe we are angels and that to do good is the chief object in our lives, with a small remuneration thrown in, to which we scarcely give a thought. (quoted in Reverby, 1987: 131-32)

Professionalizers deemed such bread-and-butter concerns "petty self-interest" and a "tradition foreign to the spirit of nursing." Although they too wanted higher wages and an end to student exploitation, professionalizers insisted that the status of nursing would suffer through the expression of working-class concerns such as increased salaries or improved work conditions. Hence, they focused on the culturally approved alternative: the nurse's womanly character and adherence to the service ethic.

Such a strategy created deeper rifts in the nursing profession. In addition, it fostered greater antagonism between nursing, medicine, and hospital administration. Hospital administrators were opposed to anything that might increase their operating costs, and university-educated nurses would clearly be more expensive than hospital-trained nurses. Physicians were opposed to anything that might threaten their hegemony; they wanted nurses as their helpers, not as their colleagues.

In response, the professionalizers appealed to the interests of hospital management by advocating ideas of efficiency or scientific management (Reverby, 1987). They attempted to break down, analyze, and time each step in the work process, separating conception from execution. Nursing administrators would implement the de-skilling process, gaining control over conception of the work process, and leaving staff nurses to execute it. This approach enabled proponents of nursing professionalization to redefine nursing, separating the manual from the mental tasks. They hoped that such a "scientific" analysis would justify their attempts to rid nursing of its lowly reputation as menial work.

The professionalizers welcomed support for their vision of the transformation of nursing offered by the Goldmark Report, an "objective, scientific" study on nursing education and distribution, commissioned by the Rockefeller Foundation. The conclusions of this report reflected the views of the professionalizers. It recommended high educational standards for entering nurses and the replacement of student nurses by graduates, with "hospital helpers" to carry out the routine menial duties of a "noneducational" nature. Further, the report advocated university-based schools of nursing as the training ground for the profession's future leadership. In other words, it recommended a rigid hierarchy within the nursing profession in which educated, middle-class nurses would perform the mental work of nursing, and undereducated, working-class nurses, the "hospital helpers," would carry out the more menial tasks. Class bias was written into the Goldmark Report:

These undereducated, unprepared women make trouble within the profession. Many of them are drawn from a social group which is not strictly professional in character. They are the ones talking trade unionism for nurses. It is natural that they should. Their fathers, brothers and sweethearts are ardent members of trade unions. . . .

Somehow these undereducated women, in inadequate social and academic background, must be kept out of the profession. Fortunately there is no longer any need for them. . . . Therefore, our first problem. . . . How can women be kept out of nursing who manifestly have not the proper background to enter?" (quoted in Reverby, 1987: 176)

Left entirely out of this picture were the private duty nurses, graduates of hospital training schools who continued to work in the home market (even as student nurses moved into the hospitals).[7] Although they exercised greater control over patient care and were not subject to the strict discipline and poor work conditions of the hospital, the private duty nurse faced problems in maintaining a market for her services. As more patients began to use the hospitals, private duty nurses began to lose their patients to the student nurses staffing the hospital. They also faced strong competition in the private duty market from less expensive, untrained nurses. Some nurses followed their patients to the hospitals to work as "specials," private nurses in private rooms. For most, however, employment prospects became increasingly bleak. During the 1930s and into the 1940s the private duty market collapsed altogether (Melosh, 1982).

The Great Depression permanently altered employment options for private duty nurses since home care became a luxury that middle-class patients could no longer afford. High unemployment forced private duty nurses to turn to hospitals for jobs. As increased medical specialization and technology required hospital nurses to become more specialized, former private duty nurses faced regimentation within bureaucratic hospitals.

The new array of hospital techniques for both patients and nurses fostered a new role for some nurses, however: that of hospital foreman, supervising a new hierarchy of subsidiary nurses. The nursing professionalizers urged hospital administrators to hire educated graduate nurses of middle-class origins for these positions. Administrators were not hard to persuade on this point since they were able to hire nurses with more education and experience for the same wage as the student nurse, given depression-era unemployment. At first, grateful for work, graduate nurses accepted this condition. In time, however, graduate nurses responded to this situation with unrest, high rates of absenteeism, and turnover. Graduate nurses were more reluctant to take hospital positions because of overall poor conditions of work, not simply low wages:

Principally, it was because of the heavy patient load. Every single nurse said she wanted to stay in it, but, she wanted above all things to be able to give artistic nursing care to her patients, and she felt she had to neglect patients when she had a heavy patient load. . . .

It wasn't so much an increase in salary which they sought as it was an opportunity for greater satisfactions in work, opportunities to improve, recognition of service and that type of thing. (quoted in Reverby, 1982: 360)

The ANA, principally comprising nursing educators and administrators, was not concerned with organizing nurses to gain greater control over the conditions of their work with facilitating a better relationship among nursing strata. Rather, as proponents of professionalization, they were interested in enhancing the image of nursing by ridding it of the "dirty" menial tasks (later to become known as "nonnursing tasks") and its working-class members. Their goals coincided with those of hospital administrators; both sought a subsidiary nursing workforce. The hospital was interested in such a labor force because it would be less costly than the graduate nurse; the ANA saw this new stratum as a step toward elevating the status of the graduate nurse.

The ANA hoped that graduate nurses would become managers, and subsidiary nurses would perform the more menial, nonnursing tasks. Once again, however, their goals were not realized. All nurses, as salaried employees, were subordinate to the needs of the institution. Hospitals required a nursing workforce that was flexible, capable of switching nursing roles as the need arose. If patient care providers were in short supply, any nurse, foreman or subsidiary, should be able to fill the vacancy. Such blurred distinctions between nurses threatened the professionalizers' goal of a rigid, hierarchical division of labor between nurses.

Although the ANA criticized trade unions, many staff RNs and subsidiary nurses joined them. The human capital vision of professionalism began to weaken its hold as poor work conditions intensified and the conflict of interest among nursing supervisors, educators, and staff nurses became more crystallized. Letters to the editor in nursing journals of the 1930s and 1940s illustrate such heated clashes. One nurse wrote in 1945,

Phrases such as "professional prestige," "suffering humanity," "personal satisfaction" and a "grateful public". . . do not compensate for any lack in the pay envelope. No butcher has yet accepted any one of them in exchange for a pound of hamburger!

Another nurse wrote: I advise general duty [staff] nurses to leave the opiates of a super professionalism and the sentimentality of an unrealistic Florence Nightingalism to their "superiors" and get down to cases with their own interests. But don't count on the ANA. (quoted in Melosh, 1982: 199)

Conflicts between adherents of the more elitist, human capital interpretation of professionalism and proponents of the need to work continue to resonate from staff and head nurses today. Mary Ann Silver, one of the staff nurses from Mt. Zion Hospital, remarked, "Besides taking care of patients, I'm working to put shoes on my son's feet. You really lose your sense of idealism after a while. . . . Nursing administrators just don't see that I work to support my life outside the hospital too." Such a comment was just as appropriate in the 1880s as it was in 1985. The same debates still rage on.

Organizational Strategies in Nursing

Professionalization, the effort to gain monopoly control over the nursing market and educational system, is the strategy nursing educators and administrators have pursued since the 1890s and continue to pursue today. The unstated goals of this strategy are to control the supply and class background of nurses produced by the nursing schools in order to enhance nursing's social image and economic reality.

A multitude of studies commissioned by nursing organizations have legitimated this strategy (Goldmark, 1928; E. Brown, 1948; ANA, 1979, 1965) under the guise of standardizing the educational process by which nurses obtain their licensure. These studies claim that the current process "contributes to the subordination of nurses" (Sweeney, 1980). At present an RN license can be obtained in one of three ways: (1) via a bachelor's degree from a four-year college or university; (2) via an associate degree from a two-year community college; or (3) via a diploma from a three-year hospital apprentice program.

The most powerful organization promoting educational reform for nurses is the ANA, which represents approximately 15 percent of all RNs. This organization is well financed and well organized at the national, state, and district levels. With an annual payroll of over $2.5 million, the ANA employs state and national lobbyists to fight for its position on monopoly control. Hence, the tactic of professionalization involves political control outside the workplace, where battles for occupational turf and licensure are fought.

In 1965, the ANA passed a resolution to differentiate the "professional" RN with a bachelor's degree from the "technical" RN with anything less than a college degree. In 1975, the NYSNA, an ANA affiliate, pushed this 1965 proposal to its logical conclusion, passing the 1985 proposal which called for a B.S.N. as the minimum requirement for RN licensure and an associate degree as the minimum requirement for practical nursing licensure (LPN). In 1978, the ANA supported the 1985 proposal, more recently retitled the Entry into Practice Proposal.

While increased education is always, in the abstract, a laudable goal, this has been challenged by those nurses from the "wrong" background. Working nurses without the litany of letters after their name claim that mandatory credentialism has served as a form of social mobility for some and exclusion for others. It has created an elitist culture in nursing, whereby educated nurses, full of theory, are reluctant to get their hands dirty in caregiving. This problem has reached epidemic proportions in medicine, nursing's model, where physicians have been dubbed as greedy, to say the least, and are getting their hands slapped and pockets controlled by federal legislators.

Of the 1.7 million RNs, 87 percent had no university degrees in 1982 (67 percent had diplomas, and 20 percent had associate degrees). By 1989 that number had fallen somewhat for nurses, to 70 percent with no nuniversity degrees (60 percent with associate degrees and 10 percent with diplomas) (Bureau of Labor Statistics, 1992-1993). The antipathy toward the ANA proposal has clearly been considerable. Seventy-two percent of all RNs polled in 1982 were against it (Clark, 1979). Thus, the strategy of professionalization remains a viable, albeit volatile, nursing strategy.

Labor Unionism

Labor unionism has been a focus of organizational energy since the turn of the century. Organizers fought to increase control over staffing, job security, grievance procedures, autonomy, and salary. With employees arrayed on one side and management on the other, unionists saw themselves as locked in economic struggle within the workplace. Their essential tools were the right to strike or sick-outs.

This strategy is hardly new. Trade unionism spread rapidly among nurses throughout the 1930s, only to be curtailed in 1947 when the Taft-Hartly Act precluded employees of nonprofit hospitals from attaining legal protection for collective bargaining. This act exempted nonprofit hospitals from the National Labor Relations Act, which guarantees employees the right to organize and bargain collectively. In 1974, amendments to Taft-Hartly restored the same right to collective bargaining for these health care workers as those guaranteed to industrial workers.

The amendments to Taft-Hartly were pushed forward by several changes in the hospital industry, which accelerated during the 1960s. First, the increased size of acute care facilities disrupted the more personal authority previously exercised by administrators and department heads, as 2.5 million employees were added to the health care workforce between 1950 and 1970. Second, third-party insurers (both public, such as Medicare and Medicaid, and private, such as Blue Cross-Blue Shield) replaced charitable contributions and fee for service as the mainstay of hospital budgets. Hospital administrators were no longer able to dig deeper into their budgets to satisfy wage demands. Finally, the unskilled hospital workforce, previously comprising of older European immigrants, was replaced by African-Americans and Hispanic and Caribbean migrants. By the mid-1960s, nonwhites made up 75 percent of the service and maintenance workers in New York City's hospitals. These changes cemented the stratification of the hospital workforce and accentuated differences in social and economic rewards, creating fertile ground for trade unionism (Fink, 1986: 180). Registered nurses, although predominantly of European background, felt themselves to be on the short end of the hospital reward stick as well and were therefore similarly susceptible to unionism.

Nationwide, over 20 percent of all RNs belong to some kind of labor organization.[8] Forty percent are organized into labor unions (approximately 60,000 nurses). These labor unions include Service Employees International Union (SEIU), which represents 30,000; District 1199 of RWDSU, which represents another 20,000; and independent unions, which represent another 10,000.

Substantial numbers of nurses are also represented by the American Federation of Teachers (AFT), the American Federation of State, County and Municipal Employees (AFSCME), and the United Food and Commercial Workers International Union (UFCW) (Brint, 1986: 50). Thus, trade unionism remains a potent organizational strategy for nurses bent on achieving workplace security and greater authority over their working lives.

Professional Unionism

The ANA was never happy about the prospect of losing nonadministrative nurses to labor unions. Indeed, in 1946 it adopted an Economic Security Program (ESP) with these goals:

1) to secure for nurses through their professional associations, protection and improvement of their economic security--reasonable and satisfactory conditions of employment and,
2) to assure the public that professional nursing service of high quality and in sufficient quantity, will be available for the sick of the country. (Denton, 1976: 112)

Allergic to working-class unionism, these professional unions offered a sanitized alternative, a mixed strategy: one part popular individualism, where individual nurses pursue their own educational credentialism and exhibit "proper behaviors" (compliance with management), the other part involving work control tactics: economic struggle within the workplace between management and employees in the form of collective bargaining. Lest this be confused with real unionism, these organizations refrained from calling work stoppages and in fact secretly collaborated with management. Finally, and most important, the professional unions supported the ANA strategy of lobbying state legislatures for control over nursing education and practice. The structure of the professional union illuminates the seemingly contradictory tactics it employs. The professional union (known as the Economic and General Welfare division), is a department within the State Nurses' Association (SNA), which is an affiliate of the ANA. These state nursing associations have boards of directors comprising primarily nursing educators and administrators. Any nurse who is a member of the state nursing association (including those ineligible for membership in the professional union) has an equal vote on any issue within the SNA's domain. Thus, nonmembers of the professional union vote on its policies and hold its purse strings.

Professional unionism solved the ethical dilemma posed by the managerial use of professionalism: that nurses must not "neglect" patients for their own "self-interest" as employees. Nurses who bought into this form of coercion, that their personal responsibility to patients superseded their rights as employees, saw the ESPs as an appropriate, nonmilitant alternative. Between 1950 and 1968 the

ANA Economic Security Program included a no-strike clause based on this personal responsibility doctrine. By 1957 43 state nursing associations had adopted the ESP, and by 1986, SNAs represented 60 percent of all organized RNs (approximately 120,000).

CONCLUSION

The economic and political processes that transformed the organization of work in the United States since the 1870s gave rise to salaried, white collar occupations. These new occupations became stratified into segments, some with greater and some with lesser amounts of control over their work. Within the nursing profession, economic and political processes divided the occupation into distinct strata with different levels of control over their different goals in the workplace.

NOTES

1. In 1860 only 15 percent of all women worked outside the home. However, their options increased over the next 50 years, especially in white collar sectors that expanded during World War I, such as the communications industry, advertising, and sales (Kessler-Harris, 1982: 224).

2. This is not to negate that such goals were shared by professional educators themselves as well.

3. To gain insight into nurses' daily lives in the late 19th and early 20th centuries, I rely on several of Reverby's (1982) vivid historical depictions derived from this period's nursing journals.

4. Of course, such work varied by race and ethnicity. Irish and black women, for example, were more likely to work as domestics, and Jewish and Italian women were more likely to be garment workers (Steinberg, 1981).

5. Middle- and upper-class women began leaving their urban and farm homes toward the end of the 19th century despite the prevalent values that dictated leisure and the absence of paid work for such women. According to Kessler-Harris, this exodus was due to a declining birthrate and technological advances, both of which lightened the middle-class woman's burden in the home. (Some, such as Schwartz-Cowan, 1983 argue the opposite: that technology in fact increased women's work.) Nevertheless, Kessler-Harris suggests that washing machines, vacuum cleaners, and oil furnaces freed middle-class women and their daughters from the household. Although many women responded to their new situation with boredom and depression, often culminating in "neurasthenia," an illness where the prescription for recuperation was to lie in a darkened room all day, others went off to newly emerging colleges and universities of the 1870s. Some went into medicine, law, and academia, but most continued to be drawn to the pre-Civil War women's associations that focused on public altruism: cleaning up prostitution, abolishing slavery, attacking poverty and poor work conditions. By 1892 hundreds of these small women's clubs joined together and formed the General Federation of Women's Clubs. These clubs pulled women into the community, fostering the development of new

occupations for themselves. New jobs opened up in the social services such as child labor investigators; others opened in journalism and nursing. Between 1890 and World War I, the number of women seeking professional training mushroomed. Between 1900 and 1910, the number of trained nurses alone increased sevenfold. In social work during the early 1890s, there were only 1000 female social workers, whereas by 1920, that number had increased to 30,000.

Although these middle-class women were entering the so-called professions, these occupations rapidly became gender divided. In both social work and teaching, for example, administrative jobs were taken over by men. Similarly, in libraries, all influential positions were taken by men, and in nursing, women became subordinate to male hospital administrators (Kessler-Harris, 1982; Stroeber, 1984).

6. In fact, by the 1890s, poor white women were being pressured into the workforce as their husbands, fathers, and brothers suffered from death and disability in the Civil War, the mines, steel mills, and the railroads. By 1890 three-quarters of all teenage girls sought wage work (Kessler-Harris, 1982; Ferree, 1987).

7. Until the 1920s, 70 to 80 percent of all nurses worked in private duty. Nursing jobs in hospital administration and public health were restricted to nurses with more education or with diplomas from elite nursing schools (Melosh, 1982: 77).

8. While one mights be tempted to assume that gender is an important variable here, since historically women have been less likely to organize than men, in fact, Freeman and Leonard found that the female portion of all union members increased from 19 percent in 1956, to 36 percent in 1984, to 58 percent in 1990 (Milkman, 1993). And among white collar workers, because women predominate, they constitute 61 percent of those unionized. A significant caveat here, however, is that these authors do not differentiate between trade unions and professional unions in the data. Unionism here includes such professional associations as the National Education Association and nurses' professional associations (Freeman and Leonard, 1987: 191).

Chapter 3

Nurses' Class Position

Given the different types of white collar workers that have emerged since the end of the nineteenth century (the high level, highly educated wage earner; the low level, moderately educated wage earner; and the independent professional entrepreneur), the question arises: What is the real class position and class identity of this stratum, and where do nurses, as white collar professionals, fit? This becomes a significant issue as one attempts to grapple with the divergent views and actions exhibited by white collar workers. For example, controlling for race, union membership, religion, age, family income, region, and gender, 47 percent of "upper" white collar workers (professionals and managers, according to the U.S. Bureau of Labor Statistics categories) voted Republican in the 1988 election. In comparison, only 27 percent of the "lower" white collar workers (clerical, secretarial, and sales workers) voted Republican in the same election (Halle and Romo, 1991). Using such U.S. Bureau of Labor Statistics classifications to evaluate voting data and, ultimately, worker attitudes obscures the segmentation within groups of workers. Nurses, for example, call themselves professionals, yet some are high-level managers, some are mid-level managers, and some are simply direct care providers. In which Census Bureau category should they be placed?

This chapter addresses this question by clarifying that each occupation actually comprises different class positions, which cross-cut the boundaries of white collar, blue collar, and U.S. Bureau of Labor categorizations. Delineating these class positions provides a better understanding of the varied class identities and actions in evidence today.

There are three general positions on this issue: (1) those who argue all white collar workers are subject to common processes of proletarianization (such as de-skilling and loss of autonomy) and thus identify with the working class (Braverman, 1974; Derber, 1982; Mallet, 1975; Gorz, 1972); (2) those who argue white collar workers are subject to common processes of professionalization (with increased control and power over their work and in society in general) and thus identify with the middle class (Bell, 1973; Friedson, 1973a; Ehrenreich and Ehrenreich, 1979); and (3) those who argue white collar workers are subject to processes of both proletarianization and professionalization and hence identify, in a contradictory manner, with both the working and the middle classes (Lederer, 1967; Corey, 1935; Oppenheimer, 1985; Wright, 1976).

The third position best represents white collar workers and nurses specifically. The other two positions are simply too general. Some white collar workers experience proletarianization, some are professionalized, and some simultaneously straddle both processes of proletarianization and professionalization. Such coterminous trends of professionalization and proletarianization occur not only between white collar occupations but within them as well. Within the same occupation some segments experience a tremendous loss of autonomy, some experience greater control and power at work, and some experience trends in both directions at once. We need to take a more critical look at the way we use broad categories based on occupation or industry, since the categories themselves are a source of confusion.

E. O. Wright spells out this notion most clearly through his concept of contradictory class locations. He argues that the traditional three Marxist categories of class--bourgeoisie, petite bourgeoisie, and proletariat--are contradictory class locations: managers, partial managers and supervisors, semiautonomous employees, and small employers. These class locations are differentiated by each group's different levels of control within the process of production, causing them to be objectively segmented, preventing them from sharing one class position. This contradictory position prohibits a unified white collar vision, even when divided into upper and lower distinctions, and prevents them from aligning with either management interests or working class interests as a whole. In addition, it precludes a unified consciousness based on occupational similarity.

Wright offers a powerful framework for understanding objective formulation of contradictory class locations. He argues that class position is determined by differential levels of control in the labor process and has articulated three of them: the economic, the political, and the ideological. Economic control refers to decision-making authority over who produces what, or control over the division of labor in the workplace. Political control refers to the power to determine the fate and daily work life of workers in a supervisory hierarchy. Ideological control refers to how a product is produced: can workers exercise independent judgment over both conception and execution in their work, or are they subject to de-skilling, a separation of conceptual work from its execution?

These three levels of control in any given organization determine the class position of its workforce according to Wright. In an ideal model, these levels of control can be mapped onto traditional categories of class analysis: bourgeois, proletarian, and petite bourgeois class position. High levels of economic, political, and ideological control would indicate bourgeois class position and low levels of economic, political, and ideological control would indicate a proletarian class position. In the same ideal model, petite bourgeois class position would be determined by high economic and ideological control although no political control, since most petite bourgeois (small business owners for example) have few or no employees over whom political control can be exercised (Table 3.1).

Wright argues however, that this is only an ideal model. In reality, most workers have varying levels of economic, political, and ideological control. Class position is thus not a static category. Rather, it is one in which individuals occupy ambiguous or contradictory class locations, somewhere between or within two categories. Hence, contradictory class locations are those that hover near the boundaries of the working or ruling class.[1]

TABLE 3.1
Processes Underlying Class Relations

ECONOMIC OVER OWNERSHIP (control over investment and accumulation process)	CONTROL OVER PHYSICAL MEANS OF PRODUCTION (what is produced)	CONTROL LABOR POWER OF OTHERS (how it is produced)
Bourgeoisie +	+	+
Proletariat -	-	-
Petite bourgeoisie +	+	-

Source: Wright, 1976: 75.
Note: + plus: high control;   - minus: low control

Wright's model is structural; it is not about the subjective experience of class (contradictory or otherwise). However, it has considerable potential for explaining variations in political consciousness or collective strategies. I utilize Wright's theory on contradictory class locations for that express purpose: to correlate it with subjective class identity and collective actions (in Chapter 4), as it provides an excellent model for understanding that ambiguous strata of contemporary white collar workers.

EXTERNAL CONSTRAINTS ON CLASS POSITION

Models of class structure cannot be applied in a historical vacuum. For nurses, the politics of health care economics has been a profound source of constraint on their efforts to organize and prosecute collective interests.

Between World War II and the mid-1970s, federal support for health care skyrocketed, and incentives for reducing costs were minimal. In the 1940s, the federal government sent an infusion of funds into medical research and training, as newly developing medical technology began to be viewed as an important component of America's international technological strength. Hospital construction and expansion projects also benefited from federal largesse because of its potential for creating employment. Most important, by 1965, Congress and President Lyndon Johnson established Medicare and Medicaid after long-felt pressures from labor and senior citizen constituencies.

Expenditures in these areas soared until the 1970s when ominous declarations of a health care crisis were sounded. Health care costs totaled $69 billion in 1970, jumped to $230 billion by 1980, and soared to $800 billion by 1993 (Starr, 1982, 1993). The federal government bore an increasing share of this burden; its portion spent on health care rose from 2.6 percent of total outlays in 1965 to 37 percent in 1970. By 1980 federal health expenditures were 9.1 percent of the gross national product, and by 1992, they had reached 14 percent (Starr, 1993). If the system were to continue with its current policies, health spending in the 1990s would jump to 30 percent of federal spending, according to the Congressional Budget Office (Starr, 1993).

Some attributed these rising costs in health care to Medicare (which in 1993 paid for 90 percent of reported hospital costs alone), Medicaid, and expensive scientific advances. Others argue they resulted from the structure of medical financing itself. Indeed, many suggest that an incentive system to encourage higher costs is actually built in. Both patients and providers are insulated from the true cost of treatments since third parties (private insurers and government) pay approximately 80 percent of the cost. Doctors and hospitals are reimbursed by these third parties on a fee-for-service basis and earn more income as their volume of services increases. Hence, providers have an incentive to provide an ever greater number of services. Because providers are reimbursed on the basis of their costs, the greater their costs are, the greater are their reimbursements. Spiraling medical inflation ensues.

Managed competition has been put forward by the Clinton administration as the salve to such spending, which if left unchecked, would increase an additional 1 percent of the GNP every 35 months (Starr, 1993). While there are several alternative proposals on the table for managed competition, (from John Garamendi, California's insurance commissioner; the Jackson Hole group led by Alain Enthoven and Paul Ellwood; the Conservative Democratic Forum in the House of Representatives; and liberal Democrats such as former senator George Mitchell), the basic proposal involves the development of regional groups that would purchase health insurance as a cooperative. These purchasing cooperatives would contract with a variety of health plans, each maintaining a minimum, standard benefit package.

The cooperatives would acquire their revenue from a variety of sources (still a matter of intense debate). Employers, employees, individuals with greater ability to pay, and government would most likely all contribute. The purchasing cooperative would pay each health plan a standard rate, based on the lowest premium, adjusted for average risk of the enrollees. Government would subsidize the unemployed, thus creating universal health coverage. A federal health board would oversee the entire process: set standards for coverage, monitor outcomes of treatment, and regulate the flow of funds into the purchasing cooperatives and out to the health plans (Starr, 1993: 44).

While the jury is not yet in on the outcome of these proposals, certain changes in health care over the last decade have already produced tangible results. In 1983 Congress came up with a prospective payment system in the hope that fixed costs would control medical prices. This system placed a ceiling on total Medicare payments for a given service, regardless of actual cost. It also incorporated an incentive system for cost control: when services are delivered at costs below approved rates, providers keep the difference. If a hospital or doctor exceeds the top price for a particular service, it has to absorb the cost. A series of 487 DRGs were established by the Health Care Financing Administration, an arm of the Department of Health and Human Services, for determining payments. For example, if a patient is diagnosed as having lung cancer, the provider will be reimbursed for so many x-rays, biopsies, chemotherapy treatments, and so on. This system seems to have reached some of its desired effect since the rate of increased Medicare outlays dropped from 20.1 percent in 1979-80 to 6.3 percent in 1990-91 (Marmor, 1993: 56).

Although this system of DRGs is only a decade old, some of the general effects on the health care system are clear. Barbara Melosh documents four major areas of impact. First, hospitals have become acute care facilities, caring only for the sickest patients. Because of the high cost of inpatient care, hospitals discharge patients as soon as possible and simultaneously, reduce the overall number of beds. Second, hospitals have developed highly sophisticated computer systems to keep precise accounting of costs and payments and use these data to determine which types of cases (patients) are most "favorable" (profitable). Third, in their effort to cut costs further, hospitals have centralized their services, contracting out for services from one large national company rather hiring their own workers or buying from several different local companies, as was common in the past. Housekeeping, laundry, and food services can all be purchased from one central firm now. Finally, hospitals have carefully scrutinized their staff for budget cuts. (See Table 3.2 for across-the-board staff decreases in 1985.)

Medical economists predict that such trends as these will intensify if the managed competition proposals of the Clinton administration become law. As hospitals are drawn into managed care networks, they will continue to be pressured into further cost cutting, more wards will be shut down, and hospitals will merge or be closed entirely (Kerr, 1993: 11).

Because nursing services are the largest single expense in a hospital's budget and two-thirds of all practicing RNS are employed by hospitals, nurses are clearly affected by the financial restructuring that has already occurred and promises to continue in the future. Both St. John's and Mt. Zion hospitals have experienced the ripple effects of cost containment. The two hospitals evidenced several (sometimes contradictory) trends affecting nonmedical staff: (1) upgrading the nursing staff to an all-RN staff while simultaneously de-skilling them (by expanding their duties to include less skilled tasks, previously performed by housekeeping, technicians, aides, and LPNs), (2) rehiring and retraining laid-off LPNs as RN turnover rates increased due to overwork, and (3) increasing the numbers of lower paid workers (e.g., radiation therapy technologists, pharmacy technicians, and nurses' aides) to perform those duties previously performed by LPNs and nursing aides.[2] (See Table 3.2.)

Substituting lower-paid workers for higher-paid nurses, a more traditional form of cost cutting occurred in most hospitals following World War II (Table 3.2). By the mid-1960s, unskilled nursing aides constituted the largest single nonmedical hospital occupation in the country (131,000). In combination with LPNs (59,000), the aides and LPNs comprised a workforce that was more than twice as large as the RN labor force of 88,000. Other low-skill, low-wage occupations were large as well, such as maids and porters (63,000) and kitchen helpers (38,000) (U.S. Bureau of Labor Statistics, Industry Wage Survey, 1963: 2). Licensed practical nurses, aides, and various other forms of health care technicians performed many tasks currently performed by RNs today. In New York City in 1957, for example, 70 percent of the nonmedical hospital workforce was unskilled. By 1970, the majority of the nonmedical labor force was still unskilled (59 percent), but it had been reduced (Fink and Greenberg, 1989: 3).

A major cost to the hospitals of the substitution approach was increased trade unionism among the hospital's auxiliary workforce. In 1961 3 percent of all hospitals had at least one or more union contracts. By 1975 this had increased to 19.8 percent.[3] Increased unionism meant greater unrest and a demand for increased wages and benefits for members. Trade unionism, in combination with fervent lobbying on the part of the nursing professionalizers, most notably the ANA, as well as the development of more sophisticated medical technology, shifted the nursing workforce toward a higher proportion of RNs. Between 1968 and 1979, the percentage of hospital RNs increased from 33 to 46 percent. By 1982 RNs constituted 60 percent of the total hospital nursing workforce, with aides and LPNs comprising 20 percent each (Moses and Levine, 1983: 475-494). Ten years later, RNs constituted 66 percent of hospital nurses' workforce (U.S. Bureau of Labor Statistics, 1993).

With the onset of DRGs and the increase in acute care patients, hospital administrators leaned more toward hiring all RN nursing staffs. Because RNs have more training, they have been perceived as more skilled and therefore more

TABLE 3.2
Changes in Hospital Nonmedical Workforce: 1957-1985, New York City
(Number of Workers in each Category)

	1957	1960[a]	1976	1981	1985
NURSES					
Director of Nursing	141	---	142	107	102
Nursing Supervisor	1,171	1,049	1,660	2,040	1,732
Head Nurse	2,202	2,182	3,834	3,955	3,471
Clinical Specialists	---	---	110	645	270
Nurse Anesthetist	---	---	298	278	256
Nurse Practitioners	---	---	---	---	153
Nursing Instructors	455	---	331	375	334
General Duty Nurses	10,846	5,724	18,204	23,382	24,383
Practical Nurses	10,917	5,767	6,994	6,236	4,829
Nurse's Aide	10,208	13,865	17,231	13,746	14,020
TECHNICIANS & TECHNOLOGISTS					
Diagnostic Med. Sonographer	---	---	---	85	100
EEG Tech.	---	---	---	86	98
EKG Tech	---	---	---	496	394
Lab Tech.	---	---	---	1,077	885
Medical Tech.	1,315	---	1,934	2,642	2,322
Nuclear Medical Tech.	---	---	---	226	201
Radiation Therapy Tech.	---	---	---	---	99
Radiographers (X-ray)	610	248	1,175	1,448	1,253
X-Ray Supr.	74	---	212	108	129
Surgical Tech.	---	---	812	968	789
THERAPISTS & SOCIAL WORKERS					
Occupational Therapist	---	---	167	370	353
Physical Therap. Supervisor	---	---	---	92	93
Physical Therap.	372	---	367	704	678
Respiratory Therapist	---	---	472	961	662
Speech Therapist	---	---	817	153	122
Medical Social Worker	531	---	919	1,164	1,381
Psych. Social Workers	---	---	334	648	267

TABLE 3.2 cont'd

	1957	1960ª	1976	1981	1985
OTHER PROF. & TECHNICAL					
Dietician	519	392	617	672	596
Med. Librarian	—	—	90	68	50
Med. Record Administrator	—	—	177	209	154
Med. Record Technician	134	—	127	512	583
Pharmacists	—	—	736	1,082	1,083
Pharmacy Tech.	—	—	—	387	322
NONPROF. HEALTH SERVICES					
Psychiatric Aides	—	—	5,395	4,714	861
Ward Clerks	—	—	1,639	2,967	2,471
Cleaners	—	—	8,976	8,889	7,609
Maids	2,931	4,823	—	—	—
Porters	3,860	3,206	—	—	—
Kitchen Help	4,906	4,630	—	—	—
Food Service Helper	—	—	6,511	5,374	4,458
Food Service Supervisors	—	—	301	361	283
Laundry Workers	511	—	161	1,136	659

Source: Data derived from Industry Wage Surveys, Bureau of Labor Statistics, Dept. of Labor. (1957, Bulletin 1210-16, Tables A1 & A3:4-6); (1960, Bulletin 1294, Tables 5-17:13-25; (1976, Bulletin 1949, Table 1:11); (1981, Bulletin 2204); (1985, Bulletin 2272 Table 4:17-21)

ªThe data for 1960 are not as complete as the other years. Blank spaces for this year should not be construed as nonexistent jobs.

valuable. They are seen as highly flexible in their ability to perform a variety of tasks. (This has actually de-skilled RNs--in the sense that they must once again perform more low-skill tasks, not in the sense of separating conception from execution of tasks.) Hospitals have therefore chosen to replace the greater numbers of less trained auxiliary workers with fewer numbers of more highly educated RNs. A study of 118 nursing administrators in 1984 indicated that two-thirds of these administrators were shifting to an all-RN staff. At the same time, 40 percent of them were cutting RN positions, and 53 percent were cutting aide and LPN slots (*American Journal of Nursing*, 1983: 1165). This strategy has been viewed by hospitals as more desirable than hiring cheaper nursing workers. Presumably they are getting more value for their dollar.

The unforeseen cost of this approach to hospitals has been tremendous work overload and therefore labor turnover of RNs, once again increasing the threat of unrest, unionism, and increased wages. There is evidence that these new costs to hospital administrators have resulted once again in a shift of the ratio of RNs and auxiliary workers. Specialized, lower-cost technicians (pharmacy technicians) are, for example, replacing higher-cost RNs in some instances. In other instances, the threat of higher-cost specialized technicians (e.g., emergency medical technicians) also exists to replace high-turnover RNs.

Profound changes in the structure of health care financing have had a direct impact on the nature of nurses' class positions. The degree of economic, political and ideological control they exercise on the job is intimately related to these (and other) external constraints, as I will demonstrate below. Uncertain of their future and remembering their past, the nurses I talked with reflected the tension and ambivalence that has accompanied the turmoil in the health care industry.

LOW CLASS POSITION

Nurses who occupy a class position at the low end of the control spectrum are characteristically weak in the extent to which they exert authority over the economic, political, and ideological decisions that shape their work. They cannot truly influence the division of nonmedical labor, supervise other workers in the hospital hierarchy, or exercise independent judgment over both conception and execution of their tasks. Staff and head nurses I interviewed at Mt. Zion and St. John's hospitals provide useful examples.

Hospital staff nurses provide bedside care, carrying out the medical regimen prescribed by physicians. They are generally assigned to one area, such as surgery, pediatrics, or intensive care, although they are frequently floated--moved to another unit to fill in as the need arises. Seventy-nine percent of all nurses employed by hospitals are staff nurses (U.S. Bureau of Labor Statistics, 1992-93).

Head nurses (retitled senior clinical nurse and nursing care coordinator, but for simplicity's sake I will stick with head nurse) provide patient care but are also task supervisors. They plan work schedules and assign work tasks to staff nurses, LPNs, and nurses' aides, and arrange for appropriate training, on top of providing bedside care as well. They are overburdened by extensive coordination activities, ensuring that appropriate records, equipment, and supplies are maintained and available. These coordinators of nursing care have no sanctioning authority and comprise 11 percent of all RNs employed by hospitals. Both staff and head nurses are eligible for membership in collective bargaining units (U.S. Bureau of Labor Statistics, 1981; Brint, 1986: 48).

Economic Control

Staff and head nurses have negligible control over the division of health care labor, the economic aspect of production according to E. O. Wright. They are not entitled to make decisions about which tasks they themselves will perform on either a daily or a long-term basis. The spectrum of their responsibilities is completely determined for them.

Ruth Jones, a staff nurse from the general medical unit at Mt. Zion Hospital for the past 19 years, is a single woman living in a Mt. Zion-owned apartment, reminiscent of a college dorm, where other Mt. Zion Hospital workers live and socialize. Her whole life revolves around the hospital. She has seen different health care occupations come and go, many taking over what were once nursing tasks, leaving nursing with the less skilled, more menial duties in patient care:

When I started in 1969, we had 8 to 10 patients each . . . no time to even *talk* to the patients we were so busy. Since then they've hired more nurses and started to give some of our [skilled] jobs away to other departments like pharmacy and respiratory therapy.

Now . . . we've given too much away. I used to do what the respiratory therapists, social workers, pharmacists and dieticians do. . . . Five years ago there was a nursing shortage and the pharmacists started preparing medications and distributing them to the units. It did free us to do other things at the time but it remained like that *after* the shortage. *They* continue to prepare chemotherapy, and *we* hang it up and regulate it now. *They* review with the patient how long to take the medications and teach them about it . . . we don't review with patients any more.

During the shortage we did all the menial things like bed baths, dressing changes, and enemas. . . . The thing is, we *still* do these things!

Ruth Jones describes the way in which staff nursing work has been degraded over time (20 years) in ways that working nurses have not been able to stop. With each nursing "shortage," other occupational specialties have emerged and taken over work previously performed by staff nurses at Mt. Zion. Medical technicians, social workers, and respiratory therapists all gained a foothold in the hospital, picking up the slack that nursing left behind. (These occupations made inroads across the nation. Respiratory therapy for example, like nursing, joined the credentialing bandwagon, requiring formal education and licensure to practice. The average wage is $12.60 per hour, and the future job prospects are rosy, given the aging population and the increased incidence of AIDS, often involving respiratory problems [U.S. Bureau of Labor Statistics, 1992-93].)

In 1980, Mt. Zion Hospital administrators were still referring to nursing shortages, which they claimed had reached 100,000 nationwide. The hospital claimed that the nursing crisis justified the creation of satellite pharmacies. Consequently, pharmacists were hired to work on nursing units, preparing drugs and IVs for patients. The hospital also hired unit managers to lighten the paperwork load of staff nurses. These were all previously nursing duties

(Archives, Medical Staff Letter, October 1980), which nurses did not willingly give up. Although staff nurses can afford to lighten their workload, they would like to choose which of their duties they yield to others.

Because none of these specialties wants to be left with low-status tasks, which may or may not involve autonomy and creativity, occupational turf wars ensue, involving struggles between the educational and/or administrative arm of different occupations for a piece of the health care pie. Conducted outside the workplace by professional associations and, ultimately, at the state legislative level, these battles pit occupations against each other in attempts to gain exclusive licensure to practice a circumscribed nonmedical domain.

The state nurses' associations in Iowa and Ohio, for example, have fought in the state legislatures to restrict the practice of emergency medical technicians (EMTs) to nonhospital settings because they often cover temporary shortages of nursing staff. The state nursing associations fear that hospitals may begin substituting these EMTs for RNs (Melosh, 1986: 157), especially since accredited educational programs for EMTs were developed in 1982 (Institute of Medicine, 1983). Losing turf to another occupation is a threat to the integrity and economic security of an occupation's position within the health care labyrinth.

Liz McConnel is a staff nurse from St. John's Hospital who has worked in the emergency room (ER) for six years. She is personally caught up in one of these turf wars between nursing and paramedics, who in this case earn more than the RNs. McConnel describes herself as a hard worker, derived from the values she inherited from her immigrant Scottish parents. Although she is conscientious and has put in her time with the ER, she is afraid of losing her job. She has a high school diploma and an associate degree in nursing, and feels her job is in jeopardy because of the creation of this new ER occupation, the paramedic.

Others on the ER nursing staff also speak derisively of the paramedics, whom they see as having taken on the airs of macho, Sylvester Stallone types. With sirens blaring, the EMTs rush to the scene of the accident, clean up as much blood and guts as they can, and then speed over to the ER, "expecting the sea to part for them." According to the ER nurses, the EMTs treat nurses as their subordinates, rather than the other way around.

Since technological advances have virtually transformed ambulances into mobile intensive care units and EMTs are now trained in such high-tech, intensive care skills as defibrillation and endotracheal intubation, nurses are afraid that paramedics will render them useless in the ER. Although most paramedics still have less training than nurses, they earn more than nurses, most likely reflecting gender based wage discrimination. McConnel offers this interpretation of the situation:

There's a new movement going on to replace emergency room nurses with paramedics. It all started with the nursing shortage. We've now got these "Hollywood oriented types"; we call them the "Hollywood boys." They're all men and they think they can *save lives*, like on TV . . . ya know all the action at the scene of the accident. . . .

The trouble is, they want nurses to do all their schlep work . . . the bed pans etc. Well, I'll tell you, I'm not here for their schlep work.

They've had only nine months' training and make more than I do. There's nothing they do that we can't, but we do a lot more than they can.

Yet another example of such occupational turf wars involves a dispute over the development of a position known as the registered care technologist, again developed to alleviate the shortage of nurses, estimated at about 300,000 in 1988 (*New York Times*, June 30, 1988). This new category of worker would receive 2 to 18 months of hospital apprenticeship training under the arm of the state medical boards (out of the ANA's grasp) and would carry out functions traditionally performed by less skilled nurses: routine patient care such as patient temperatures, changing bedpans, and administering medications. The ANA vehemently opposed this proposal, taking the public position that it duplicates the job of nurses' aides and poses a danger to patients. But once again, the underlying issue for the ANA is that its monopoly control over patient care activities would diminish if another nonmedical, ancillary worker is created, trained, licensed, and monitored by physicians.

These occupational turf wars reflect the low economic position of staff and head nurses. While changes in health care financing are swirling around beyond staff nurses' reach, these turf wars affect them daily. Staff nurses have no real voice in the political arena where these battles are fought, since they are dominated by professional associations, the insurance industry, and state and federal government. Those nurses who do enter the fray are primarily non-direct care providers (nurse educators, administrators, and professional lobbyists), who do not truly represent working nurses' interests.

Staff and head nurses have a minimal voice in the professional nursing associations since, as low-paid nurses, they generally do not have the time or money to travel around the country to lobby state and federal government. Nor can they afford the astronomical annual membership fees ($200,000-400,000) in the organizations that sponsor professional conventions. As a result, working nurses are kept out of the dialogue, and their workplace concerns are rarely topics on conference agendas. Instead, conventions are dominated by policy matters of interest to the nursing elite (educators and administrators): credentialism, increased nursing turf, and economic and social mobility for nursing.

Joanie Williams, a staff nurse at Mt. Zion Hospital who is an outspoken African-American woman from a small town in Georgia, has thought long and hard about these issues. She initially came to work at Mt. Zion as a nurses' aide, like many other poor African-American women who came to northern cities looking for work. It took her 16 years, but she worked her way up to an LPN, then an RN, and now feels that she needs a bachelor's degree to survive as an RN. Nevertheless, she has little patience for the elitism she hears expressed by the nursing administrators and educators at Mt. Zion.

Williams attended an NYSNA convention in Albany, representing staff and head nurses from Mt. Zion. She went intending to discuss labor issues, such as staff-patient ratios, treatment of staff by administrators, and separating the union from NYSNA. She found her agenda was unwelcome and her reputation maligned before she even opened her mouth. Word had spread that Mt. Zion staff nurses were trying to decertify the professional union and were characterized as militant, irresponsible troublemakers. Williams was surrounded by nurses who, in E. O. Wright's terms, occupied a high class location (administrators and educators) and had an entirely different set of priorities. Like their predecessors a century ago, these professionalizers were still trying to separate the wheat from the chaff, in class terms. They wanted to eradicate the working-class element from the profession of nursing and focus on loftier goals of higher education. Williams said:

I went to the convention in Albany with all these nursing administrators and educators. It was like in the movies . . . they smeared us. They said we were the bunch coming to disrupt the convention and they scared everyone about us. . . .

First of all, we asked them why they couldn't hold the convention in New York City, not Albany, since 80 percent of the membership is located in New York. They told us they wanted it near the "seat" of government. Then I brought up the issues of staff-patient ratios built into the contract and that we wanted the union part of NYSNA separated from the association. . . . They looked at me as though I just fell out of a pink cloud.

Their goals are not for us. Its for themselves. . . . They don't care about the day-to-day problems in nursing. . . . They just want to *expand* the body of knowledge, *expand* the role of nursing. What body of knowledge? *What* role? *I want to do hands-on care.* With a master's degree, who you gonna put your hand on?

The ANA's overall game plan, fostered by the NYSNA as well, was to replace existing LPNs (who typically have no more than a high school diploma) with college-educated RNs in order to upgrade the occupation's status, decrease the total supply of staff nurses, and thereby increase demand (Dolan, 1979b: 519).

The supply has indeed diminished, yet this strategy has backfired to a large extent. Nursing is threatened on all sides by the emergence of new auxiliary health care specialties. Hospitals have benefited in several ways. Competition between professions generally ensures less unity between them in lean times and therefore less strength. In addition, by supporting the route of credentialism, hospitals can end up with a nursing workforce that is more educated and in theory less inclined towards unions. Further, RNs are licensed to practice more tasks for the same overall price as LPNs, once all the factors are considered. Upgrading the employee population is a widespread practice utilized by hospitals in the attempt to diminish unionization among staff (Lockhart and Werther, 1980).

The elimination of LPNs began in earnest in 1980 at St. John's Hospital, despite the fact that these nurses had, in many instances, worked there for over 20 years. Patty Cilantro, director of continuing education (and a member of the hospital administration), supported this move for nurses at St. John's. She grew up in a small town in upstate New York as the daughter of a foreman. He was in charge of the loading docks at IBM, always considered a blue collar job by his company. She worked at the loading docks herself during the summers and felt the sting of humiliation, since her father was never considered a white collar worker. This personal pain motivated Cilantro to become a white collar worker, no matter what the obstacles. She worked as an RN for 10 years, and then came to New York City, hoping to earn good money as a professional. She worked her way up to nursing administration, and met her husband-to-be, an investment banker with a new job at Goldman and Sachs. Their joint family income would exceed $150,000 as long as he survived the Wall Street layoffs of the late 1980s. She desperately sought the prestige afforded by the professional titles and income bracket they would enter. She felt nursing could achieve this prestige if hospitals hired all RNS, and she wanted to be a part of such a movement:

I was interested in an all-RN staff. Get the biggest bang for your buck. . . . A higher level of practice. You want the highest qualified resource. I can have two RNs for the price of three LPNs before. The bottom line is, college-educated RNs should mean more status, more respect for nursing, and for all of us.

The same type of nursing workforce can be found in other parts of the country as well. In Indiana, for example, one state nursing association official noted that "135 nurses' aides positions were just eliminated in one stroke, [which] means of course, that RNs are now doing all of the aides' work" (*American Journal of Nursing*, June 1983: 864).

The total nursing staff at St. John's was cut, and, as in Indiana, RNs were left with responsibility for the entire spectrum of nursing work, previously shared with LPNs and aides. The increased responsibility enlarged the RNs' share of less skilled bedside care, such as provision of bed baths, enemas, and bedpans, generally referred to by professionalizers as nonnursing tasks. The staff RNs, exhausted from overwork due to an inadequate labor force, had little recourse other than to withdraw their labor power by quitting, not striking. When they did so, the hospital responded by rehiring and reeducating many of the previously laid-off LPNs. Thus, although the RNs lack real economic control in the workplace and lost the battle, they can sometimes win the war. The hospital did hire more staff.

Theresa Robinson, a former LPN at St. John's for 13 years and a staff RN for the last 5, went through the layoff and rehiring process. Although she was happy to have a job 13 years ago, having just arrived in Brooklyn as a single black mother from rural North Carolina, both her attitude and her work title changed over the years. Her actual work, however, remained about the same:

In 1968 LPNs were head honchos around here. . . . We had a lot more power than LPNs have now. We could order supplies, do the budgeting . . . initiate treatments, give cardiac resuscitations, and administer emergency drugs. We did patient histories, nursing assessments, drew bloods. . . . First they started taking away our tasks; then they took away our jobs. It made you go from bein' somebody to feelin' like you were nobody.

The hospital decided it wanted all RNs. Sixty-eight LPNs and 42 nursing assistants were laid off. In place, they hired 40 RNs.

The doctors relied on a lot of us LPNs. After four months they called us back. They *begged* us to come back! The RNs just didn't want to do the work we did. They were quitting. The hospital forced us to come back. You'd be automatically cut off from your unemployment if, after the third call, you didn't come back to work. They notified unemployment about the job openings.

It was a depressing three months. I lost 78 pounds. . . . Most of us went on to college to become RNs. The pay is slightly better, $3,000 more. . . . But to tell you the truth, in the actual things I do, it's the same as the LPNs. There's no difference.

Robinson was caught between a rock and a hard place. The content of her LPN job dwindled until it was finally eliminated. Then she was forced to come back as an RN, doing more work with fewer staff and a minimal increase in compensation. Staff nurses had negligible control over this. The hospital shuffled its people and job categories like a deck of cards in order to maximize its economic benefit, an effort that was triggered by declining federal support for health care.

Staff and head nurses lacked workplace control over these work categories and staff changes. In E.O. Wright's terms, they occupied low economic class positions since they had no direct influence over the division of labor. Only indirectly, through high quit rates, were they able to influence change.

Another example of their low economic class location is reflected in issues surrounding staff-patient ratios, a crucial workplace issue for bedside care providers. The ratio of medical and nonmedical staff per patient changes each day and is recalculated daily as the number of patients changes. A central administrative office exists solely to determine the number of nursing staff that will be deployed on each unit, based on a daily patient census (number of patients) and their acuity levels (level of illness). Using such calculations, nurses are floated (moved) to different units as the need arises, regardless of their expertise.

The process of floating further diminishes nurses' control over which tasks they will perform. For example, if, on a specific day, central administration determines that there are not enough staff nurses in the labor and delivery unit, a staff nurse who has practiced in the oncology unit for 20 years might be floated to labor and delivery, regardless of experience.

Sam McLaughlin, a head nurse at St. John's Hospital, described one such floating experience she had. She is a single woman from a small town in Long Island who has been practicing nursing for 30 years. She was floated to labor and delivery recently, after having been away from the department for 15 years:

I was with an ulcer patient, and someone ran in the room and said, "quick, go into the delivery room: there's no nurse in there." So in I went even though I hadn't done a delivery for 15 years.

"MASH" [the television series] is the closest thing to reality in nursing there is. The patient was out [unconscious] for her C-section, and the doc insulted the nurse on duty. She weighed about 400 pounds, and he said to her, "Ruth, please move your breast. I can't see what I'm doing."

She ran out of the room crying down the hall, and they tell me, that's when they came for me.

McLaughlin's description lends a bit of drama to the issue of floating, but it is real nonetheless. Staff nurses' duties are redefined for them as a regular part of their day, as the need arises. Nancy Jefferson, a seasoned staff nurse for the past 10 years at St. John's, described rather matter-of-factly how her tasks change, bordering on the illegal at times, based on the availability of medical staff at any particular moment.

We put patients on monitors, give vaginal exams, and deliver the babies. . . . I've actually done lots of deliveries. Its not legal, but if there's no doctor around, what are you gonna do? Even if there *is* a doctor around, they usually just stand there at the foot of the bed and catch the baby as it flies out!

Nursing work also changes according to the time of shift worked (day, evening, or night). Each shift has a different number of auxiliary staff employed, and the tasks that nurses perform vary. There are fewer workers on the night shift than there are during the day. Therefore, nurses who work at night perform a greater array of tasks (regardless of whether they are licensed to practice these tasks) than those working during the day. An oft-repeated phrase in nursing is, "An LPN is someone who does at night what the RN does during the day." And an RN is someone who at night might do what LPNs, respiratory therapists, inhalation therapists, and even physicians do during the day.

A head nurse from Mt. Zion who has worked the evening shift for the past five years explained this discrepancy in nursing based on work shift. John Turbett is a self-described aspiring "yuppie" from Schenectady, New York, who went into nursing because it guaranteed him a job right out of college. In addition, as a male, he felt assured that job mobility to the top of the nursing administrative ladder would be a breeze. He described the evening shift's division of labor as quite different from that of his colleagues on the day shift:

I do chest physical therapy in the evenings which only pulmonary therapists do during the day. We just don't have any of the therapists here on eves and nights. . . . LPNs do everything I do except start IVs or add meds to them, which just changed recently. Before, they did the same, if not more than I. . . . We just don't have enough RNs.

Thus, staff and head nurses are up against several factors that prohibit them from controlling the division of labor, or having economic control, in Wright's terms. On both a daily and a long-term basis, they are compelled to respond to changes in their work tasks imposed on them by actors both outside and inside the workplace. External forces, such as contracting fiscal resources, changes in health care financing, and the maneuvering of professional associations, undermine their leverage over the division of labor in the hospital. Internal factors, such as the time of shift worked and the hospital's attempts to shuffle jobs and staff-patient ratios, also detract from their level of economic control.

Ideological Control

Staff and head nurses also suffer from low levels of ideological control: discretion over how they do their work. They lack the authority to make independent judgments or decisions over how they ought to deliver patient care or pace their work. Pam Mahoney is a staff nurse who has worked at Mt. Zion for 19 years. As the daughter of a coal miner from the small town of Kingston, Pennsylvania, she always knew she wanted to leave her home town. Few of the people from Kingston earned over $10,000 a year, and the occupational hazards of coal mining were all too common. Her first job in Kingston was at a large sewing factory, where most of the town's young women worked after high school. She earned $3,800 for her first year. Taking a rather brave step, she moved to New York City and became a nurse, an occupation her family perceived as safer, cleaner, and more respectable. She described her earliest years of nursing at Mt. Zion as similar to her industrial seamstress work; nursing was factory-like in its regimentation:

When I first came to Mt. Zion I worked under an English head nurse. . . . With her, everything had to be exactly the way she wanted . . . even how the water pitcher should be carried. Each water pitcher had to be carried *individually*, from each room on a tray, no carts . . . and you had to keep upright, your back perfectly straight. . . . She would inspect our beds, watch you strip it, and then make it, with the patient in it. Everything had to be absolutely perfect; no wrinkles.

Today, staff nurses would most likely not be disciplined for poor posture, and they work with highly advanced technical equipment, yet they are still subject to control over how they provide care. Staff nurses cannot, for example, adjust the oxygen levels for patients with pulmonary fibrosis (a lung disorder that in its last stages, can make patients feel they are drowning), even if that patient is suffering from excruciating fear and requests more oxygen. They are afraid, understandably, that making such an independent decision would get them fired. Pam Mahoney explains that staff nurses are not allowed to help such patients even if their lives depend on it:

The staff nurses won't touch the oxygen levels, no matter what the patient wants. . . . They're afraid of losing their jobs. They read what's on the chart and just do what the doctor orders. They can't respond to the individual situation and think it through.

They're not allowed.

   Their frustration and lack of input in defining and executing patient care stem
from two factors: (1) nurses' subordination to a multilayered hospital administration and (2) nurses' subordination to physicians.
   Ronnie Blevins is a colorful character with a quick wit who elaborated on these
issues. She is a clinical supervisor who has worked at Mt. Zion Hospital for 23
years and was late for our meeting because she was attending her hospital aerobics
class, jumping, twisting, and turning with plumbers, orderlies, aides, and social
workers to the tune of Tina Turner. Born and raised in Longfield Hill (in Kent,
England), a village with a total population of 60, and common-law wife to a
prominent Mt. Zion physician, Ronnie Blevins seems to enjoy class leveling
situations, such as the aerobics class where everyone from janitors to middle
managers sweats it out together. She also takes a certain defiant pride in being
labeled "only a nurse," a comment she hears time and again at dinner parties she
attends with her physician husband. She says she loves her work and claims only
a job as a chorus girl could lure her away from nursing. Nevertheless, Blevins is
well aware of the drawbacks in nursing and describes the way in which hospital
administration robs staff nurses of independent judgment. Nurses must perform
each task according to predetermined hospital regulations. Each hospital has a
book of nursing rules the size of a Manhattan telephone directory, delineating in
painstaking detail how each nursing task must be carried out. Deviations from
policy can, and indeed do, cost nurses their jobs:

See this stack of papers? [She shows me a stack five inches thick.]   These are guidelines
on nursing care, which I have to learn and pass on to my nurses . . . for giving an enema,
making sure siderails are up, how to give an IV. . . . When a nurse does *any single* thing
in this hospital, even giving a bed bath, there are guidelines on *how* to do it, and she
better follow them.
   If you had a headache, I'd need an order, from an intern who may be one year out of
med school, to okay a Tylenol.

   Betty Jean Alario, a staff nurse from St. John's Hospital's ICU for nine years,
also described the detailed rules nurses are required to follow. She believes nurses
are so engrossed in following rules that they seldom have enough time to provide
adequate care for their patients. She went into nursing straight out of high school
because it was an altruistic job available to women, where she could help people
and collect a steady paycheck at the same time. (Her husband became a policeman
in Brooklyn for similar reasons.) In her early years as a nurse, she said, she was
"laid back," happy to get paid for helping people. As time went on, she began to
realize that she was unable to provide the quality of patient care she was capable
of giving because of the bureaucratization of hospital nursing. She began to lose
patience with the seemingly senseless bureaucracy, in which independent judgment
became a thing of the past:

There is no patient care people can give today. Anyone who tells you that, it's a crock. You're so busy making sure you follow all the rules: that I took my vital signs every two hours, documented that I did or did not give the meds . . . and signing everything you did. . . .

We're constantly documenting, documenting, documenting. . . . There's just no time to care for the patient. If I were a patient in these conditions, I know the first thing I'd need was a shrink consultation!

This is why so many nurses just come in to work, don't look at anything, and leave at 3 p.m. They don't want to do anything that will make them lose their jobs.

Having to break the rules in order to provide adequate patient care was a continual refrain heard from the nurses I interviewed. Jenny Cornwell, a staff nurse at Mt. Zion for nine years, described a situation in which she was forced to employ her own judgment, despite rules to the contrary, in an emergency situation:

If I followed all the rules and "didn't think" like I'm supposed to do, I'd leave nursing. If you really care for your patients, there comes a time when you have to act. You can't worry about being reprimanded for not following the rules.

You know, like in [the film] *Terms of Endearment*, when Shirley MacLaine started screaming down the hall, "Why does my daughter have to wait until 10:20 to get her pain killer when she's in pain *right now*?" Well, those are the kind of rules I'm talking about.

I had an epileptic patient once, who started to get the tremors. I knew in a few minutes he'd be shakin' all over, and the whole bit, so I called for an attending to give him the meds. No answer, for 40 minutes, then an hour. Meanwhile, my patient is going into convulsion. Finally, after waiting for over an hour, I started my own IV, which only the docs were supposed to do. The other nurses were having their own seizures when they saw what I was doing. But I did it for the patient, because I knew what I was doing. I've been working with these patients and my attending [senior physician] for years; I knew he'd back me up. . . .

Well, it turned out all the doctors were having a conference and weren't answering any calls. When the attending finally showed up, he actually thanked me.

Jenny Cornwell is a self-described maverick who has been told by her superiors on several occasions not to rock the boat. "The boat was already rockin'," she says, but they continued to move her from department to department to prevent her from rabblerousing. In this case, the physician supported her independent decision, but the norm in these situations is one of top-down authority. While patients want assurance that some form of procedure is followed, the rigid rules dictating every aspect of how nurses do their job is overkill, epitomizing nurses' low ideological control.

Subordination to physicians is another exasperating aspect of nurses' lack of input into job procedures. Physicians are notorious for rarely sharing information with nurses on the specifics of their patients. Nurses are therefore often unable to make informed decisions or are prevented from doing so. As Cornwell explains: "One physician I used to work with would say to me, 'Don't think. Just don't think. Your job is to do what I tell you and that doesn't require you to think.'"

Such comments confirm the abundant waste of nursing talent, all in the name
of maintaining a stratified workforce, upheld by de-skilling. Etha Henry, a 27-
year-old staff nurse who had worked as an army nurse before coming to the
neonatal ICU at Mt. Zion six years ago, expressed a similar sense of uselessness.
She feels her years at Mt. Zion Hospital have turned her into a "worker," a cog in
a machine, deprived of creative or independent thought. According to Henry, the
unspoken assumption at Mt. Zion is that nurses are insignificant helpers, and
should be discouraged from expressing their own ideas. Most physicians, she
feels, block nurses from exercising any intellectual independence.

I was an army nurse for three years and had more autonomy than I do here. . . . If I have
a suggestion on how to do something a little better at this hospital, the physician says,
"*Are you challenging me*?" . . . No one wants your input at this place. You're encouraged *not* to speak up. . . . You're not important here as a nurse; your input is valueless.

Thus, the profession of nursing, as far as staff and head nurses are concerned,
in reality has few of the independent characteristics professions are supposed to
possess. They are in fact constrained by bureaucratic procedures and rules that
govern most aspects of the delivery of bedside care.

Political Control

Wright's model of contradictory class locations posits a third dimension:
political control, subordination to a rigid supervisory hierarchy that dictates
preformulated rules over work time, place, and behavior. Nurses in a low class
position are a case in point. They are severely restricted in their work behavior,
and they have minimal breathing space when it comes to work habits. (This is
reminiscent of Richard Edwards's notion of bureaucratic control, in which workers
are subject to stringent written rules governing their work tasks [Edwards, 1979:
ch. 8].) Staff and head nurses are subject to supervision in the form of these
written rules, enforced by physicians, hospital administrators, and all nurses above
them in the supervisory hierarchy. While they do not actually punch a clock, they
must sign in and out, facing reprisal for arriving even minutes late to work. They
must work mandatory overtime on holidays, weekends, double shifts-and without
breaks, if so assigned. They can be floated regardless of their expertise.

Such rigid regulations governing nurses' work behavior are clearly a reminder
of the factory workplace, not the easy-going professional work environment that
nurses are supposed to find in the hospital. Jenny Cornwell describes the arbitrary
authority nurses are subjected to noting that they have no "room of their own":

Our lives are not our own. We're told *when* to come to work, *what* weekends to take off,
which holidays we get. . . . Our requests for special days are either granted or not,

according to the whim of the supervisor. . . .

Nurses have no space of their own at work. I can't even say this is *my* desk or *my* chair. They'll float you any time.

Heather Goldblum, a staff nurse who has worked in the cardiac operating room at Mt. Zion for eight and a half years, corroborated Cornwell's description of nurses' subordination to the often arbitrary discipline of a supervisor, governed by the clock. As an operating room nurse, Heather is responsible for maintaining a sterile environment in the room, dusting, arranging the furniture, scrubbing her hands, and sterilizing much of the room itself. She greets the patients, attempting to put them at ease, and consults with the anesthesiologist, standing by in case the physicians need anything during the operation. Being married to a Mt. Zion physician, one would think Goldblum's attitudes toward the rigid rules nurses face might be somewhat muted. On the contrary, she was militant in her opposition to nurses' subordination to stopwatch techniques. She explained why she was unable to keep our interview appointment one day:

The reason I didn't call you at 11:15 today to cancel our appointment was because my *supervisor wouldn't let me out*! We work by factory rules here, ya see. . . . You have to sign in and out, get permission to take a break. . . . You have to call a supervisor anytime you want to do *anything* . . . even to make a goddamn phone call.

Most staff nurses concurred that they are treated like workers--disciplined first and asked questions later if accused of breaking the rules. Joanie Williams described one memorable occasion when she had been so disciplined by her supervisor. Her six-month-old daughter had been in the ER since 4:30 that morning with a serious asthma attack, and her child care arrangements had fallen through for the day. Finally, after several tries, she was able to round up a relative to watch her baby for the day. She was understandably distraught:

I was late, and when I walk in my supervisor screams at me, at the top of her lungs, "Don't you have a clock?"

I asked her if she was interested in *why* I was late. She didn't answer but just kept on screamin', "You're late; OR 4 is waiting for you. . . . You're going to have a meeting with the coordinator about this, and its going into your folder."

I knew she wanted to discipline me with her gang of three there against me. The supervisors try to intimidate you. They gang up against you in a group: two supervisors, one coordinator, and you, a staff nurse. You are put on the hot seat. . . . Most people give in. They expect you to shut up and do as you're told. Not me. I was furious after all I had already been through.

Such insensitivity seems to come with the territory--the bureaucratization of hospitals, where individuals become "OR nurses" or "EMTs," who have to make their quota of patients for the day, pushed on by layers above them. Everyone is simply following the rules, with no time for personal mishap.

Head nurses enforce such rules as well but are, ironically, also subject to them. One would assume that head nurses have greater political control because they exercise a modicum of authority over others in the supervisory hierarchy. Nonetheless, they remain in a low class position because the type of political control they have is only to coordinate nurses' work rather than to issue sanctions. They are in fact bound to adhere to the same rigid rules as those they must enforce with subordinates.

Carla Johnson used to be an LPN; she went to college and worked her way up to RN and now head nurse, earning a slightly better salary. She started a master's degree in nursing management but quit because, as she put it, she "didn't like learning how to manipulate nursing staff for management's ends." Carla has worked at Mt. Zion Hospital for 12 years and now, as head nurse, feels caught in the middle:

The hospital wants us to be management. . . . They *tell* us we're management. . . . We're expected to be both management and staff at the same time. I do patient care, and, I'm in NYSNA; but they want us out of it.

Management says your goal as a manager is to meet the needs of the staff . . . but, as staff yourself, you know you can't give that kind of freedom because you just don't have the coverage.

I can't increase my staff. If I get a sick call, I'm responsible to make up staffing with what I've got . . . and not accept unsafe staffing.

Management tells you, "Be flexible with their mealtimes, or let people come in a bit late.". . . But [having been] staff, you know nurses can't leave a patient. . . . Someone has to be there at the assigned time.

Despite a glimmer of supervisory power, head nurses are basically controlled by rules defined from above. They assign work shifts and mealtimes yet cannot sanction others for infractions, and they subordinate themselves to an array of superiors. This contradictory class location (vis-a-vis the political level) is reflected in the comments of Robin Mintener, a black woman from the industrial city of Birmingham, England, who has worked as head nurse at St. John's for six years.

My role is dual. Sometimes I don't have any authority whatsoever. Like I can't counsel, suspend, or interview a nurse. Yet I'm supposed to "facilitate between the nurse and physician."

I'm non-managerial, but I don't do only manual work either. I'm responsible to supervise and direct, but also do patient care.

They tell me my position is important. To me, it's not. Its just a title without power or authority.

Mintener can exercise minimal control over others yet is subordinate herself to an institutional hierarchy. Administration flatters her with inflated notions of her position, but given her actual work, she knows she has great responsibility without authority. Rules originate from higher up in the authority structure, giving head nurses the appearance of control but negligible amounts in reality.

Overall, staff and head nurses are in a low class position. They must salute and adhere to a rigid set of rules handed down by a variety of supervisors in the medical, nursing, and hospital administration hierarchy. Genuine authority is simply a mirage, contributing to their low political control. They cannot determine the division of nursing labor since it is subject to external forces, such as changes in health care financing, occupational turf wars, shift time worked, and hospital manipulation of job classifications and numbers of personnel per patient. Finally, they have minimal ideological control over their work lives since they must adhere to strict policies governing each component of care they provide. These low levels of control contribute to their overall low class position, which in Wright's model places staff and head nurses close to the boundary of the working class.

MEDIUM CLASS POSITION

Professionals who occupy a medium class position have greater authority within the supervisory hierarchy and are able to exercise more independent judgment in their work. However, they, too, like those in a low class location, have minimal control over the division of labor in which they are embedded. This is what E. O. Wright's contradictory class location really refers to: workers who resemble the working class in some areas of work and management in others.

Nurses in this class position include those from Mt. Zion and St. John's hospitals with such job titles as clinical supervisor, coordinator of nursing, nursing educator, nursing care coordinator, and clinical nursing supervisor. None of these job positions are eligible for bargaining unit status because they all fit within the National Labor Relations Board (NLRB) purview of "supervision within the interests of the employer." This means that any employee who hires, fires, disciplines, and evaluates the work of others must be excluded from the bargaining unit (Lockhart and Werther, 1980: 16). Such supervisory nurses comprise 5 percent of all hospital nurses (Brint, 1986: 48). I refer to these supervisory nurses, minimally involved in the provision of patient care, as middle managers.

Economic Control

Like their counterparts in low class positions, middle management nurses have no leeway in devising their own position within the division of labor. Clinical supervisors from Mt. Zion Hospital provide the clearest example of this lack of economic control, since their jobs have been reclassified by hospital administration. At the same time, however, some of the external forces that affect the low economic control of staff and head nurses (occupational turf wars, staff-patient ratios, and time of shift worked) have had little impact on clinical supervisors.

Clinical supervisors manage nursing on the units. They prepare monthly time schedules, budgets, and staffing needs, and they audit quality assurance documentation. In addition, they hire, fire, discipline, and evaluate their subordinates. These truly managerial duties render clinical supervisors ineligible for bargaining unit status.

Ronnie Blevins, the clinical supervisor from England who has "gone a bit batty [from] having worked at [Mt. Zion] for too long" (23 years), provides details on her new supervisory work. She jokingly describes herself now as neither working nor middle class, but rather from the "queenly class":

I come in, listen to report from night shift or, I kibitz with my other peers in the nursing office so they don't think I'm *really* from the queenly class--or mad at them. I go in there and fight for staff, fight not to float staff, and hear what's going on in the department.

Then I rush back to my office, read the volume of mail that crosses my desk. . . . Most of my time is spent on paperwork. I plan the time schedule for 44 people: nurses, nurses' aides, unit clerks; I plan in-house classes for staff, do the budget four or five times a year. . . .

Then I go back to the unit and check on the staff, make sure they're doing their own paperwork. I review the nurses' evaluations of themselves. . . . I let them write their own because I have to hand in evaluations annually. And I do the budget, hire and fire nurses--none of which I ever did before.

Until 1976, clinical supervisors at both Mt. Zion and St. John's hospitals had the job title head nurse and practiced direct patient care, with few supervisory duties. The situation changed overnight at Mt. Zion when the hospital began juggling job descriptions in order to prevent increased unionization. Nurses received a memo from the vice president of personnel in February 1976 informing them that their responsibilities would become supervisory imminently, eliminating bedside care from their work. The change resulted from the National Labor Relations Act's 1974 amendment that removed the exclusion of voluntary, nonprofit hospitals from participation in bargaining units.

Supervisors, however, were not to be protected by the act. In the case of RNs, the NLRB found them to be supervisors only if they carried one or more of the following types of authority: "schedule employees' vacations and days off, discipline employees, assign duties to other employees, conduct employee evaluations, effectively recommend terminations, have a salary which is higher than staff nurses, attend management meetings, have their opinion given weight in hiring new employees or, authorize overtime" (Archives, Memo from VP of Personnel, Feb. 23, 1976). Clearly, the new title of clinical supervisor met these criteria.

Jean Omohundro, another clinical supervisor from Mt. Zion who lived through the sudden change in job description, discussed openly why the hospital reclassified head nurses into managerial positions. I met with her in what she called her office, a converted linen closet that was so small that I had to hold my breath in order to slide past one chair to get to the other.

In 1976 they converted our titles from head nurse to clinical supervisor: . . . One Wednesday afternoon they said to us, "As of Friday, your jobs won't exist. If you wish, you may apply for one of the available positions."

Once they changed our titles and expanded the role, they said to us, "You're management now." They did this for a few reasons. The number one reason was to get head nurses and supervisors out of the union. Unbeknownst to us, they knew long ago that this would be much too managerial for a union position.

It happened slowly. Before, I could never hire anyone. Now, I can hire whoever the hell I want. We went to court for two years to prove that we didn't meet the category for supervisors. But we didn't win. They got us to hire and fire, which is crucial for the NLRB. Anyone with critical influence on administrative decisions can't be part of a union, and we had critical influence. . . .

So, we're managers now. . . . If they want you to be middle managers, you're middle. If they want you to be upper, you're upper.

Omohundro felt trapped by her lack of economic control but chose not to leave her job, in spite of a high joint family income. After 20 years in nursing and a long court battle over union eligibility, she felt too wedded to her work.

The exact same process of forced promotions occurred at St. John's Hospital. First the title head nurse was changed to executive head nurse, and then to nursing care coordinator, once again to remove the position from union eligibility. These nurses were far from the driver's seat concerning the content of their jobs. They could not control the division of labor in which they worked. In Wright's terms, they had a low level of economic control.

Ideological Control

Although middle management nurses rank low on economic control, they can expect a greater degree of ideological control. They have greater latitude in making independent decisions than their counterparts in low class positions. They are not direct care providers subject to rigid rule books on how to provide patient care. Rather middle management nurses have the authority to conceive of and initiate changes, large and small, in the way nursing care is provided in their unit, even though they cannot execute their ideas without approval from above.

For example, Jean Omohundro was able to develop primary nursing, whereby each nurse is assigned one set of patients for whom she or he is completely responsible. Omohundro saw this as humanizing the process of delivering patient care, allowing patients to become familiar with their care providers, and nurses to see their patients as more than just "the cardiac in room 420." Primary nursing was to replace team nursing, which more or less dehumanized patients. Jean Omohundro decided along with many other nurses that team nursing treated patients too much like a slab of meat in a processing plant, and she worked to alter the organizational structure:

We were the first to do primary nursing. I had gotten some new grads who didn't like team nursing. We all sat down and decided we wanted to do primary care. So, come hell or high water, I was gonna do it, and I did. It had to get the approval of committee after committee . . . but we started the ball rolling. Later, the whole hospital followed.

Omohundro could not put such a process into action without an array of approvals from nurses, physicians, and hospital administrators above her. Nevertheless, ultimately she was able to persuade these administrators that primary nursing had improved nursing (and patient) satisfaction across the country, while minimizing employee turnover and nursing costs. Primary nursing was finally passed at Mt. Zion, much to the delight of Omohundro and her staff (Archives, Medical Staff Letter, March 1981).

Ellen Precht, a middle management nurse from New Orleans who has worked at Mt. Zion for 13 years on the psychiatric unit, was also able to improve the structure of patient care. A high school graduate with a diploma in nursing, Ellen Precht put in her time as staff RN and worked her way up to clinical supervisor. She initiated a pilot project in psychiatric nursing using a technique she had observed at Long Island Jewish Hospital: therapeutic communities, where each patient becomes a member of the unit's "community," participating in group meetings, cleaning, cooking, and other chores. Although Ellen claims that implementing her ideas required an inordinate amount of cajoling, to say nothing of committee time, she felt quite satisfied that her job innovations might eventually be put into practice.

Staff nurses praised the successful programs initiated by other middle management nurses as well. Sara Neisser, another clinical supervisor, proposed a system of pain management for cancer patients, that would enable patients, rather than doctors, to regulate their own pain medications. Previously, patients were treated for pain only at times specified by the doctors. (This lack of patient control over pain management has been a source of conflict between nurses and doctors, highlighted by Jenny Cornwell, who referred to Shirley MacLaine's anguish over her daughter's unnecessary pain in the film *Terms of Endearment*.)

Sara Neisser introduced another program of around-the-clock visiting hours, instigated by several Hasidic Jewish patients, whose relatives did not wish to leave them alone at night, in the event they died without a rabbi present. After going through the chain of command, Neisser was able to change the visiting system altogether, allowing patients' families to visit any time and sleep over if they chose to do so. These examples serve to demonstrate that middle management nurses have far greater latitude in doing their work than frontline nurses, even though they are dependent on approval from above for execution of their ideas. Their creativity is not completely squelched. Unlike staff nurses who are told "not to think," middle management nurses are allowed to utilize their brain power. The organizational structure permits these middle managers to simply care more for all concerned.

Ruth Jones, the staff nurse at Mt. Zion who has seen health care occupations come and go and nursing projects start and suddenly die over the past 19 years, takes a dimmer view of such nursing "freedom," however. To her, it is all relative. Middle managers' innovations can be overruled in a flash by physicians and hospital administrators who might disapprove of the particular proposal or the middle manager herself:

The hospital dictates how we should function and do our jobs. There is a medical board in the hospital that says how RNs should function. The vice president of nursing sits on that board, but physicians are above her. If they or Dr. Glen, the new chief executive officer of the medical center, decide against primary nursing, we don't do primary nursing anymore. Even the VP of nursing is powerless.

On smaller matters, however, middle management nurses are able both to initiate and execute their own ways of doing things. Jean Omohundro explains that units on the day shift at Mt. Zion (e.g., psychiatry, surgery, general medicine) are decentralized, each acting as an autonomous "mini hospital." The middle management nurse responsible for this "mini hospital" can determine how minor work procedures will be conducted:

The day shifts are decentralized like 20 different companies within one conglomerate. Each one functions in its own way, like individual little companies under one umbrella. Every day unit is like its own hospital--surgery, psych, they all function on their own . . . like self-contained little hospitals.

We can make our own rules; if we want to take temperatures or blood pressures once a day we can. . . . Over the minute-to-minute functioning, we have more say. Evening and night shifts are still centralized though.

Despite their ultimate subordination to various levels up the hierarchy, middle management nurses do have greater ideological control than staff and head nurses. Although they are unable to implement innovation in the nursing work process without approval from above, their overall attitude toward their work seemed to be much more positive than most staff nurses I interviewed, reflecting how detrimental a total lack of ideological control can be.

Political Control

Middle managers enforce rules from above on workers below. Of course, they themselves are subject as well to the hospital chain of command, dominated by physicians and nursing and hospital administrators. They, like thousands of other white collar workers in similar contradictory positions, are simultaneously management and employee. Yet middle management nurses have more political control than head nurses because they have sanctioning power over others: to hire, evaluate, and fire other nurses. They also dictate where and when other nurses must work, determine time off, and participate in management meetings. In contrast, head nurses are simply task supervisors, able to instruct other nurses on which duties to perform.

Mary Ellen Fein, a middle manager at Mt. Zion, is an example of the ambiguous position inhabited by clinical supervisors at the political level. She was a staff nurse for nine years and feels conflicted over the wedge that separates staff nurses from those above them in the hierarchy, including herself. Despite the fact that her husband earns well over $200,000 a year and that she lives in an exclusive neighborhood in New York, Mary Ellen Fein feels tension over her objectively contradictory class position. She is forced to dampen staff morale by floating often inexperienced nurses to patients' bedsides, due to staff shortages. Although she knows this practice can be dangerous, her own position is insecure, and she must follow orders:

As management now, I am forced to see things slightly differently--for example, floating nurses. I personally hate it. The nurses hate it. But when I get three sick calls on one shift, it's *my* responsibility to make sure nurses are there for the patients. I'm held accountable.

So I float nurses to other floors. Then people react by calling in sick more, and I have to float more. The cycle just starts going. . . . Thing is, I'd probably do the same thing they're doing if I were still a staff nurse.

Despite their apparent clout, middle management nurses are still vulnerable. Because they are no longer bargaining unit employees, they themselves can be easily fired. Ronnie Blevins, one of Mt. Zion's premier clinical supervisors, felt this job insecurity quite keenly during 1980s, a decade of hospital staff cuts:

The way they're closing units, my job security is very poor. Under current conditions . . . tomorrow I could be out.

As managers, they fire us according to how they want to. I have no recourse. The hospital gives six months' severance pay, a reference and, a sweet good-bye. They have lots of underhanded methods of getting rid of you if they want. They can say a new chief of the department is coming in and wants to hire his own senior clinical nurse. So sorry.

Job insecurity for nursing managers at St. John's Hospital is the same. "If the chief executive wants a new machine or two more physicians, they chop at nursing's middle managers, notorious for getting canned. One never knows who'll be next around here," says Patty Cilantro, director of continuing education for nursing.

Nurses in this medium group occupy the most contradictory class position of all nurses. Although they have minimal control over the division of nursing labor--little economic control in Wright's terms--they have considerable control over the ideological and political aspects of their work. They are able to suggest and initiate new ways of doing work in their units, a source of great satisfaction to workers who have this freedom and a source of major frustration for nurses who are prevented from exercising such a seeming luxury. While middle management nurses are unable to implement real change in their work without approval from above, they feel more optimistic, knowing someone will hear their case and respond, whether positively or not. Hence, middle management nurses lie somewhere between the working class and management on the level of ideological control at work. On the political level, they exercise considerable sanctioning power over others (in their ability to hire, evaluate, and fire their subordinates), imposed on them by the hospital. Yet they themselves are susceptible to the same, often arbitrary sanctions from their superiors. Their political control is muted by their own job insecurity. Their position in the political arena is highly contradictory, placing them in some middle ground, a medium class position somewhere between the working class and management.

HIGH CLASS POSITION

Nurses in a high class location, the end of Wright's spectrum, have the greatest levels of economic, political, and ideological control. They have the most control over the division of labor, the greatest authority in the supervisory hierarchy, and the most authority to exercise independent judgment in their work, compared with all other nursing segments. This does not mean, however, that they have complete autonomy in any of these areas. They do not. Although their class position is contradictory (because they simultaneously control and are controlled by others in each arena), it is not as distinctly ambiguous as that of middle managers, since these nurses are strictly administrative, with no direct involvement in patient care. Nurses in this category have such titles as vice president of nursing, assistant and associate directors of nursing, and directors of recruitment and continuing education at both St. John's and Mt. Zion hospitals. These administrative nurses are most definitively excluded from the bargaining unit and comprise 5 percent of all hospital nurses (Brint, 1986: 48).

Economic Control

Administrative nurses do not generally win occupational turf battles within hospitals alone. These battles are fought outside the hospital by professional nursing associations that lobby state and federal government. Charlotte Ramsey, vice president of nursing at St. John's Hospital, speaks about her role in these turf battles within the hospital. Ramsey is an old-timer who grew up in Tarrytown, New York, where she received a diploma in nursing after graduating from high school, 35 years ago. At that time, directors of nursing wore "Nancy nurse caps" she says and functioned in the stereotypic subservient, female role of the 1950s. They were the strong, silent types who stood up when doctors entered the room and had to use their "feminine wiles" to question doctors' orders. Today, Ramsey sees herself as a modern executive, competing with male vice presidents for power. Coyness is not on her agenda. She arrives at work at 6:30 a.m. each day and leaves at 9:00 or 10:00 p.m., in order to keep up with her workload. "Physicians," she says, "are still back in the stone ages," continually trying to overrule her decisions on the division of labor. "But, after all," she notes, dripping with sarcasm, "they're still physicians and I'm just a nurse." Charlotte Ramsey feels she loses ground if she stands still, so she pushes on to extend her domain:

The more people and money I control, the more power I have. Nurses want equality between medicine and nursing. . . . We want to make more decisions, have more control. . . . As it is, we're always stepping on what they claim is *their* turf.

We can't refer breast cancer patients to a therapy program without a physician's order. . . . We just developed a new diabetic teaching program and the physician canceled it out, saying nurses can't just implement this program without his approval.

Clearly, at this level, there is still major conflict between doctors and nurses, but the content of that struggle is light-years away from the battles being waged between staff nurses and physicians. The focus for nurses in a high class location is generally on empire building--acquiring more occupational turf to bolster their individual and occupational power base. For nurses in a low class location, the focus is primarily on improving their ability to provide quality patient care without having jobs gnawed away, piece by piece, by other medical and non-medical encroachers.

Despite these battles within the hospital (which nurses generally lose to physicians), nurses in a high class position possess much greater control outside the institution over the division of nursing labor. They are major players in the legislative arena where policy sets occupational roles. Their primary strategy is to change legislation over who does what in health care. One example of their efforts to gain greater control over what nurses do involves the fight for third-party reimbursement for services provided, the most sought-after prize in health care. As a result of heavy lobbying efforts by both the New York and New Jersey state nursing associations, each state passed laws allowing direct third-party reimbursement to nurse practitioners, certified nurse midwives, and a few nonnurse health care providers. Despite strong resistance from the AMA, patients are now billed directly by these practitioners and reimbursed for the cost (Melosh, 1986: 157). This represents a major victory in the battle for nursing turf because it permits independent nursing practice, autonomy, and fee-for-service relationships, a privilege previously enjoyed only by physicians. In contrast, the majority of nurses employed by hospitals are unable to charge a fee for their services because their work is collapsed into the overall plant costs, along with heating, lights, and housekeeping. This is a brutal reminder of their dependent status as hospital employees.

Penny McCarthy, director of recruitment and retention at St. John's Hospital, participated in this victory. Although McCarthy considers herself a member of the working class based on her $45,000 salary and was a nursing representative for the economic and general welfare department of NYSNA for seven years (the professional union), she fully believes in the need for nursing to fight medicine's monopoly in health care:

I am a delegate to the ANA and a member of NYSNA, active in shaping policy at the convention. I'm on the legislative committee where we are lobbying in behalf of specific bills. Right now we're working on third-party reimbursement for RNs outside the hospital. Nurses need to fight for themselves, fight back against physicians' control over us.

Length of stay for hospital patients is being shortened; they're going into home care now. I think this situation, if we play our cards right, will do a lot for us [nurses] economically, and medicine will have little to say about it. RNs can go into home health care and hopefully be eligible for reimbursement.

While few nurses would disagree with Patty McCarthy that nurses need higher salaries and better relationships with physicians, most frontline nurses (staff and head nurses) do not put these issues, or fee-for-service homehealth practice, on the front burner. They want personal integrity and control at work, not raw power.

Nevertheless, given the decrease in patient hospital stays due to recent changes in health care financing, many occupations are fighting for a piece of the ever growing homehealth care pie. The number of Medicare-certified home health agencies nearly tripled from 2,212 in 1972, to 6,007 in 1986, dropping slightly to 5,877 in 1987, as new restrictions on Medicare rules were implemented (Eckholm, 1993: 24). Social workers, RNs, physical therapists, and respiratory therapists, to name a few, are fighting for some of this action.

The strategy employed by administrative nurses in this fight for power involves anti-trust claims. In the case of the *Mutual Assurance Society of Alabama* v. *Federal Trade Commission* (Testimony of ANA on Reauthorization of FTC, 1983), the ANA argued that the Federal Trade Commission (FTC) must prevent state medical associations (such as the Alabama State Medical Association) from monopolizing health care practice. In fact, they had sued the Alabama State Medical Association for anti-trust violations, arguing that these associations prevent midwives and nurse practitioners from diagnosing illness and prescribing treatments.

The Alabama State Medical Association had sponsored the formation of its own insurer, Mutual Assurance Society of Alabama, which restricted nurse practitioners and midwives from independent practice, by preventing them from obtaining malpractice insurance. The ANA fought to overturn such anti-competitive market practices so that they too might have the opportunity to become independent entrepreneurs.

In short, the administrative nurses' higher level of economic control lies in their organized fight *outside* the hospital to increase their monopoly control over both the division of nursing labor and the economic rewards of independent practice.

Administrative nurses also exercise such economic control within the hospital by manipulating nursing jobs inside the institution. Although the ultimate decision on such matters rests with chief executive officers (almost always physicians), nursing administrators act in consort with their administrative colleagues in order to prove that a particular mix of staff (more RNs to LPNs, for example) is cost-effective.

Nursing journals attest to this process: "While hospital administrators are tightening their belts by laying off and reassigning staff and closing units, nursing administrators are capitalizing on the situation by changing staff 'mix': letting go of 'non-professional' nurses and hiring new BSN RNs. Increasing numbers of hospitals are phasing out nurses' aide positions altogether; some places have seen massive layoffs of LPNs and aides" (*American Journal of Nursing*, June 1983: 860).

Charlotte Ramsey, who has been at St. John's Hospital for only five years, described how she was instrumental in changing the proportion of non-RNs to RNs with college degrees:

The mix used to be 60/40 [RNs to non-RN nurses]; then we changed it to 70/30, and now it's 80/20. We upgrade positions with attrition. As LPNS and nursing assistants resign, we don't rehire at those levels. We upgrade those positions to RN--hopefully, RNs with BSN degrees.

If the 1985 proposal were passed, where you have the "professional nurse" and the "technical nurse," I'd probably reverse my ratio of professional to nonprofessional staff. . . . You'd need fewer care planners and more care givers. . . . But, right now, we need more BSNs to direct the care.[4]

These examples illustrate that in fact nurses in a high class location have greater economic control compared to nurses in low or medium class positions, and they attain such authority through extraorganizational means. They wage occupational turf wars outside the hospital to gain greater organizational control within.

Ideological Control

Administrative nurses rate quite high on ideological control as well, because they decide how nursing will be provided. Although they are ultimately subordinate to physicians and other hospital vice presidents, compared to the other nursing positions below them, senior nursing administrators have the most control over the practice of nursing within each hospital.

Mt. Zion staff nurse Joanie Williams speaks with some disdain of the control administrative nurses actually wield over patient care. She feels debased by administrators who have been removed from direct care for several years, with trails of "spaghetti" after their names, as she puts it (titles or degrees, such as B.S.N., M.A., Ph.D. and so on), yet write the great book of rules.

The average director of nursing is always "Dr." this or "Dr." that (they insist on being called "Doctor"). They are constantly coming up with new guidelines, then will quote "The Book" on the *right* way to do this and the *right* way to do that. . . . How to give an enema, the *right* way. Thing is, how would they know? You get further and further away from real nursing in administration.

Despite this cynicism from such practitioners toward administrators, the fact remains, that vice presidents of nursing, subject to constraints by physicians, exercise penultimate authority over standards of nursing practice. They determine how to do blood transfusions, whether nurses should practice primary or team nursing, and whether nurses should employ documentation techniques. Their level of ideological control is high.

One means of maintaining such elevated levels of ideological control is through a widespread managerial technique known as "patient classification," a modern form of Taylorism. Administrative nurses apply this technique of patient classification in their roles as cost cutters and in so doing remove elements of independent judgment from the work of direct nursing care providers.

Nurses on the front lines of care (in a low class location) are required to record each patient's needs and the detailed tasks they carry out in order to meet those needs. Based on these records, administrative nurses then calculate the acuity of each patient (the level of sickness). From this acuity measure, the administrative nurse determines the type of care required for each patient and the amount of time each patient should command from nurses. These calculations are used to determine the number of staff needed for each unit.

Such a patient classification system not only requires an inordinate amount of staff nurse time, which might otherwise be devoted to patient care, but more important, removes independent judgment from the individual nurse providing care and places it in the hands of administrative nurses who decide on staff-patient ratios. This modern-day health care time-and-motion study places crucial decisions on caring in management's grip, detracting from a central aspect of bedside nursing. As Campbell states, "What constitutes good enough care, previously a professional judgement, becomes established by how much staff time is available" (Campbell, 1987c: 9-10).

Melon Fisher, a coordinator of nursing at Mt. Zion for the past three years, revels in this kind of ideological control she is able to exercise over other nurses, whom she characterizes as self-aggrandizers--out to get the most resources for themselves.   She describes the Taylorized nursing process in which she participates as resulting in her considerable control over the way staff nurses divide their time:

The supes [clinical supervisors] all want more staff. They think they all have the sickest floor in the division. . . . But we have a way of checking up on them . . . the patient classification system. By using the nurses' documentation, we can compare the acuity levels of patients on all the floors and determine the number of staff we'll give them. We're basically doing away with all the LPNs and jockeying the staff we've got left . . . floating them.

Such contemporary time-and-motion studies like patient classification allow administrative nurses to remove independent judgment from direct care providers. This authority places nursing administrators closer to the boundary of the upper class at the ideological level, where they form a coalition with hospital administration, cementing the divide between nursing workers on the front lines of bedside care and nursing management in the hospital control room.

Political Control

Administrative nurses have the greatest amount of sanctioning power over all other nurses. They can ultimately veto a middle manager's decision on hiring or firing and set policies on discipline. On Wright's level of political control within the occupation of nursing, senior administrators reign supreme. At Mt. Zion Hospital, units were being closed due to increased budget constraints, and administrative nurses altered disciplinary policies accordingly. To legitimate increased nurse layoffs, they handed out more disciplinary warnings and fired nurses at an increased rate. Staff, middle management, and administrative nurses all corroborated this point. Etha Henry, staff nurse from Mt. Zion, described the general atmosphere of fear that permeated the floors:

My perception is they're giving out a whole lot more warnings for the slightest thing. Like not signing out for medication, you get a warning for that. Nursing administration is now saying that after three medical errors you automatically get fired. . . . They're rating you much more severely now. . . .   Giving out more disciplinary warnings. Everyone's afraid.

Middle management nurses described actual instructions they had received from their superiors to increase disciplinary actions. Ellen Precht, a middle management nurse at Mt. Zion Hospital, explained that nursing administration instructed her to invoke a new, invisible form of control: the search for "quality nurses." The problem with this, she says, is that it is completely arbitrary. A physician may choose one individual as a "good nurse," while another physician may deem her or him inferior. "Quality" nursing is too often defined by the eyes of the beholder:

Discipline gets more rigid. . . . More people get fired. One way to fire them is to get them on discipline.

I've been to many meetings where administrators tell us you have to look for "quality." If you look for "quality" you'll naturally find a lot of deadwood out there too. Deadwood you have to get rid of. You don't keep the one who can't take as many patients as the next nurse. . . . Staff are fired this way.

This invisible form of supervisory control invoked by administrative nurses is called quality assurance, another managerial technique in which nurses are required to document every detail of their work on a daily basis, ostensibly to ensure "quality care." Nursing administrators use this technique to kill several birds with one stone; by maintaining such records on nursing care, they will not only reduce staff but will also demonstrate and legitimate the importance of and ultimately the need for, independence in nursing, lending further support for third-party reimbursement for nursing service. This system of documentation also enables administrative nurses to deflect blame from the conditions of work (e.g., staff shortages) onto individual nurses for specific infractions. Supervisory control is facilitated as each nurse documents her or his work and is held accountable for her or his actions, rather than the hospital or supervisor.

As Campbell points out, quality assurance systems defer blame from the organization and its mangers when untoward incidents happen. Detailed recording nurses are required to identify the individual nurse and her or his actions. She or he remains responsible for *actual* outcomes of care, in whatever work conditions exist. If a mistake has been made or the nurse had to skip certain tasks because of a large number of patients (to improve hospital productivity), she or he becomes personally liable (Campbell, 1987ab).

Quality assurance is an invisible form of supervisory surveillance that contributes to administrative nurses' high political control, placing them very close to the boundary of the upper class. Despite their power, however, they still occupy a contradictory class location on this level, because they, like the entire nursing cadre beneath them, are vulnerable in their own job security.

Nevertheless, nursing administrators still maintain have the greatest level of supervisory authority within hospital nursing. They determine work behaviors of nurses below them through such measures as increased disciplinary actions, firings, and invisible forms of control like quality assurance. These practices facilitate their administrative job of cutting staff to meet budget constraints and uphold their place at the wheel, steering their political authority in some directions of their own choosing.

CONCLUSION

Nurses have long been thought of as a single occupational group. This chapter should make clear that the workplace lives of modern nurses are highly differentiated. The nursing profession, along with other white collar occupations, is not one monolithic group but rather a highly segmented one, with wide variations in levels of control and autonomy.

Nurses in low class positions have little power economically, ideologically, or politically. They are white-collar employees who share the plight of the working class.

In high class positions are the administrative nurses who control their colleagues and enjoy influence outside the hospital. They share many of the powers and privileges of professionals.

Placed in a contradictory class position are middle managerial nurses. They find themselves pulled simultaneously in two directions: by forces of professionalization from above, by forces of proletarianzation from below.

NOTES

1.   As Wright states, "Contradictory class locations are variable rather than all or nothing characteristics. . . . Certain positions can be thought of as occupying a contradictory location around the boundary of the proletariat: others occupying a contradictory location around the boundary of the bourgeoisie" (Wright, 1976: 74-77).

From here on, I will refer to such class positions as simply high, medium, or low, depending on their levels of control, bearing in mind that all are contradictory.

2.   Although I wanted to examine change over time in the workforces at St. John's and Mt. Zion, these data were not made available to me.

3.   Regionally, hospital unionism tends to be more concentrated in the Northeast (New York, Connecticut, and Massachusetts), on the Pacific coast (California, Oregon, and Washington), and in the Midwest (Minnesota and Michigan), plus Hawaii (Miller, 1979:30).

4.   The 1985 proposal was a resolution passed by the ANA in 1965 calling for the bachelor's degree as a requirement for entry into nursing practice by 1985. Recently the ANA set 1995 as the new target date for this credentialism in nursing since the previous date has come and gone with its goal unmet (*American Journal of Nursing*, 1984:832).

Chapter 4

Visions of Professionalism: A Window on Class Identity

E. O. Wright's class model is valuable as an analytic tool to measure dimensions of control within the workplace. However, culture is also a critical part of the picture, and it is not addressed by this framework. Culture involves subjectivity (values, beliefs, and interpretations) and practice (rituals and collective patterns of action). It is ambiguous, full of contradictions and varied interpretations of the same event. Culture is not so much a single phenomenon as what Clifford Geertz terms "systems of interacting symbols, patterns of interworking meanings" (Geertz, 1973: 207). This chapter seeks to explain the context and patterns of varied cultural meanings found among hospital nurses. It attempts to understand the ways in which "sociopolitical thought [and actions are] bound up with the existing life situation of the thinker" for nurses (Mannheim, quoted in Geertz, 1973: 194).

Although class position does act as a powerful determinant of the subjective views and behaviors of nurses, it does not tell the whole story. In nursing, an important role is played by interpretations of individual professionalism.

Professionalism, as it permeates American culture in general, and professional schools and hospitals in particular, conjures up wholesome images of expertise, autonomy, and altruism (Wilensky, 1964); it carries a sense of unquestionable social and economic superiority of white collar over blue collar workers. Such professionalism has been historically symbolized by the physician, who (at least until recently) was thought to possess autonomy, specialized knowledge, altruistic service, and rapid social mobility. There are also other concepts of professionalism. Taken together they shape an ideology. Though nurses, self-described occupational have-nots, strive toward what they perceive as the prize in American society, true professionalism, they understand this goal in different ways.

Eighty percent of nurses in a low class position construe professionalism as work control (control over the conditions of their work). Seventy-six percent of nurses in a medium class position define it as a combination of work control and popular individualism (achieving personal freedom via credentialism) and 60 percent of the nurses in a high class position define it as capitalist individualism (gaining maximum power and profit via market control over the occupation and individual credentialism).

The process of ideological formation for nurses regarding professionalism has been one of "confrontation, negotiation and redefinition," a process that historian Sean Wilentz also found among 19th-century American artisans and entrepreneurs regarding the concept of "republicanism" (Wilentz, 1983). According to Wilentz, established principles of the Republic included notions of equal rights and virtue. But as class differences began developing between artisans and entrepreneurs from the 1770s through the 1820s, disparate interpretations of republicanism evolved as well, expressed in various forms of ceremony and ritual.

Entrepreneurial visions of republicanism stressed the notion of equality in terms of individualism: equality of opportunity, whereby each individual has the freedom to compete and reach his or her own innate potential. Failure to succeed according to this view is due to individual lack of virtue (e.g., drunkenness). In contrast, artisan republicanism focused on ideals of virtue in terms of cooperation and fraternity. Their notion of equality referred to that between individuals, diminishing the gap between the rich and the poor in a critique of the inequities of capitalism.

It is within the context of Wilentz's analysis on the formation of the ideology of republicanism, where "old ideas are re-articulated and transformed into different class perceptions," that I similarly evaluated nurses' interpretations of professionalism. Just as artisans and entrepreneurs developed entire worldviews or ideologies around their class interpretation of republicanism, so too did nurses, around the concept of professionalism.

Ideologies, as Clifford Geertz suggests, are "most instinctively, maps of problematic social reality and matrices for the creation of collective conscience" (Geertz, 1973: 220). Similarly, I suggest that nurses employ concepts of professionalism to define their "problematic social reality," which, as Geertz continues, functions to make "an autonomous politics possible, by providing the authoritative concepts that render it meaningful" (Geertz, 1973: 220). Thus, class-based visions of professionalism serve as a rallying point for nurses' class-based collective actions.

The traditional 19th-century professional, while possessing wholesome attributes of autonomy, expertise, and altruism, was also an independent entrepreneur, upholding notions of meritocracy and individualism. As class differences evolved within white collar occupations, this traditional configuration of the professional became the locus around which three different ideologies developed, each claiming the mantle of professionalism. These three worldviews have enabled nurses with shared experiences to coalesce and organize collectively around their symbols, value systems, and goals. Professionalism thus mediates between class position and choice of collective strategy, cementing nurses through shared meanings, interests, and interpretations of their experiences.

As Gramsci states, ideology acts to "arouse and organize . . . the collective will." It acts as a cement for social relations, binding individuals to one another and connecting their immediate experiences to each other (Gramsci, 1971: 126). Burawoy, paraphrasing Marx, adds to this statement: "Lived experience produces ideology. Not the other way around" (Burawoy, 1979: 17-18).

Hence, professionalism as an ideology acts to cement nurses together in each class position, giving rise to some form of collective identity and action. In addition, nurses' differential relationship to this ideology has provided a window through which I was able to peer, shedding light on some of the processes of class identity formation.

Nurses in a low class position reshaped the traditional notion of professionalism to mean work control, or greater control over the conditions of their work. They believe that professionals maintain control over their own labor by exercising independent judgments in their work, over such elements as number of staff and amount of time required for delivery of quality care. They also uphold aspects of traditional professionalism: that hard work and service to others is noble and deserving of accolade. What they reject in that traditional notion of professionalism, however, is an assumption of moral superiority, built on the competitive principles of meritocratic individualism, whereby individuals are deemed responsible for their own destiny (Newman, 1988). This is antithetical to their belief in the original version of the Protestant ethic, which suggests that hard work to benefit the community is a virtuous activity. Thus, professionalism is reshaped by these nurses into an ideology of work control, in which nurses with skill, knowledge, and devotion to service feel they deserve what is rightfully theirs: dignity and greater control over their own destiny at work.

Nurses in a low class position perceive the nature of conflict as that between management and employees at work, in their struggle for autonomy, respect, and reward. Out of this worldview emerges cooperative tactics of economic struggle in the workplace, such as collective bargaining and work stoppages (strikes, mass resignations, and sickouts), to achieve their vision of professionalism. This reinterpretation of professionalism is expressed through the strategy of trade unionism (which, of course, is abhorrent to those who define professionalism by its very rejection of such tactics). The collectivism inherent in trade union activity is indicative of at least a basic class consciousness not found among nurses in the higher class locations.

Nurses in the medium class position have reshaped professionalism to mean both work control--greater control over the conditions of their work--and popular individualism--increased status as the path to greater personal freedom from economic, ideological, and political constraints in the workplace. According to

Herbert Gans who coined this term, "popular individualism is a search for personal freedom from unwelcome cultural, social, political and economic constraints, and also, from a lack of economic and emotional security" (Gans, 1988: 2).

Drawing on a belief in the culture of meritocracy, nurses in this class position pursue credentialism as the means to attain their higher status. Based on their perceived merits (innate ability and credentialism), these nurses feel deserving of greater prestige and see themselves as superior to blue collar workers who lack credentialism and "proper behaviors" (a willingness to compromise with management). Based on their hard work and devotion to service, they also believe that as true professionals, they deserve greater discretion in the workplace (e.g., more autonomy, as well as improved bread-and-butter rewards such as higher salaries, better benefits, and greater job security). To achieve this true professionalism, nurses in the medium class position pursue individualist solutions. They believe it is incumbent upon individuals to improve their own human capital and upon the organization to recognize and reward their higher status as professional workers.

For these nurses, workplace conflict is understood not so much as a competition between management and nurses but rather as a competition between nursing and other occupations. The tactics that emerge out of this ideology involve partial use of economic struggle within the workplace (organizing among themselves to protect their workplace interests, since they are too managerial according to the NLRB decisions, for eligibility in a collective bargaining unit). In addition, they support political struggle at the level of the state, waged by nurses in the high class location, who lobby state legislatures for monopoly control over nursing markets and education. Professionalism for these nurses is expressed through a strategy of professional unionism, which they endorse and promote, although they themselves are ineligible for membership in its bargaining unit.

Finally, nurses in a high class position interpret professionalism as synonymous with the pure individualist interpretation: capitalist individualism. According to Herbert Gans, who also coined this term, "capitalist individualism is a pursuit of profit maximization, market control, risk taking, escape from government regulation, and the notion that everyone can be successful" (Gans, 1988: 2). These nurses believe individuals should take personal risk and responsibility for improving their lot in life. Credentialism and demonstration of proper behavior (compliance with the goals of hospital management) are seen as the best individual means to attain the fruits of high position. Market control over the occupation, in which nursing takes the reins (through lobbying government) and acquires a monopoly over its own schools and markets, is viewed as the most important collective strategy to achieve these individualist goals. The strategy should ultimately trickle down, benefiting individual nurses by limiting entry into the schools and the occupation. Limits at the portals of nursing should, according to this view, ideally decrease the supply of nurses, then increase the demand, and finally, reward nurses with greater status and income. This is the strategy of professionalization that perceives conflict in the workplace as that between occupations rather than between management and employees (Larson, 1977, 1980.)

Control over conditions of work such as labor shortages, understaffing, layoffs, increased workload, and overtime without pay is viewed as the individual's own problem, solved individually, by enhancing one's human capital and escaping into positions of higher authority. Losing one's grasp over these conditions is perceived as the individual's own fault, due to a dearth of ability or credentialism.

The last two variations of professionalism, popular individualism and capitalist individualism, are both intimately linked to the culture of meritocracy, a powerful thread in American work culture, whereby individuals are seen as rising and falling in accordance with Social Darwinist principles: only the strong survive. This notion embraces the Calvinist precept that God rewards the virtuous, and hence, the successful are virtuous (Newman, 1988). All participants in the marketplace are viewed as equal in their opportunity to succeed, akin to Wilentz's 19th-century entrepreneurs' depiction of equality.

According to Gans, popular individualism is in fact a logical response to the economic and emotional insecurity faced by middle Americans in a period of economic decline (Gans, 1988). Whether we view individualism as naked greed or a rational response to economic decline, the vision of professionalism embraced by nurses in medium and high class locations reflects the individualist cultural principles of Social Darwinism.

Professionalism as work control is also rooted in the cultural tradition of individualism, but it confronts the inherent contradictions of this tradition and rejects its current configuration. This vision recognizes the disparities between owners and workers in the capitalist enterprise and that the meritorious activities of hard work, altruism, and expertise, once considered valuable attributes in the construction of a virtuous society, are not necessarily rewarded. Professionalism thus signifies different worldviews or cultural meanings for nurses in each class position, reflected by their endorsement of different collective strategies. The data gathered from St. John's and Mt. Zion hospitals demonstrate that nurses in each class position reshape the ideology of professionalism according to their own class experience in the workplace, which coalesces into class-based collective strategies.

LOW CLASS POSITION

The majority of nurses in a low class position reject the traditional ideology of professionalism, which incorporates principles of capitalist individualism and the culture of meritocracy. Eighty-four percent of these nurses have come to understand professionalism as work control--the exercise of discretion over their work process. Altruism, expertise, and autonomy are part and parcel of this interpretation as well, with improved bread-and-butter issues such as fair salaries, job security, and benefits, as the just rewards for their "virtuous" activities. These frontline nurses are struggling to be professional as they define it yet know they are not. They generally experience their work as blue collar, and themselves as workers, despite the organizational and occupational rhetoric to the contrary.

Despite their training, the years of experience under their belts, and their commitment to patients, they still find themselves having to "go through a chain of command every time they have to go to the bathroom." They feel they are "treated like children, [and] deprived of adulthood" in the hospital. Despite their white collars, many want to call a spade a spade, and go from there.

Carrie Gelfan is one of the staff nurses who unabashedly calls herself a worker because she, and her school psychologist husband, have to "work from paycheck to paycheck to meet their monthly bills." Despite their education levels (he has a master's degree, and she is 12 credits away from a B.A.), she feels greater affinity as a nurse for blue collar workers than white collar:

Nurses have to stop viewing themselves on such a high pedestal just because they tell us we're "professionals."

We are salaried workers, with a little more knowledge, a little more education . . . [but basically] the same as a man who punches a time card in a factory. . . . I love my patients but . . . like it or not, we work; we are workers.

Another staff nurse who has worked in the renal treatment (hemodialysis) unit for the last eight years at Mt. Zion similarly challenges the assumption that nurses are white collar. Like most of the others, altruism is the guiding light for Ruth Jones. She wants to affect her patients not as simply "cases" but as "whole persons with lives outside the hospital as well as inside." She has attended patients' weddings and funerals, has helped them through crises, and has tried to keep up with magazines that offer the latest in counseling techniques. Yet despite her devotion to service, she knows her work is primarily manual and rhetorically asks how nursing can be considered a "profession" with the blue collar manual labor it entails.   Knowing full well how physically exhausted she is at the end of each day, she notes the irony that nursing management considers the occupation white collar, despite the mostly manual labor involved:

We're a profession? That's what they tell us. What other profession do you know that does heavy manual labor? We lift, we carry, we run, we make beds. . . . We do hard physical labor, but they call it a profession.

These nurses do not accept the cultural contradictions they face. They believe in the meritorious activities of their hard work, altruism, and expertise yet want freedom from autocratic control at work, input into the decision-making process, and improved bread-and-butter rewards for their competence.

Nurses in a low class position also bitterly reject professionalism as a form of managerial control, used to salve the wounds and inflate the egos of hard-working nurses. Heather Goldblum, a matriarch of sorts known for imparting her wisdom to neophyte nurses, is cognizant of the managerial double-speak about professionalism that nurses endure. While labeled high-status, white collar workers, she too characterizes herself as a worker, subject to factory regimentation, given her lack of autonomy as a nurse, despite her college education, and her husband's status as a physician.

Nurses want to view themselves as professionals. They don't want to be considered workers, but of course we are, and I try to tell them how we work by factory rules here: signing in, signing out, having to call a supervisor every time we want to do anything—take a break, go to the bathroom. . . .

I believe professionalism involves participatory management.

Even though, by accepted standards I'm probably considered to be in the upper class (my husband earns over $150,000), I don't deal with that class socially. I deal with other people more like me.

In addition to articulating a class identity that is distinct from her husband's, Goldblum distinguished between her own class interests as a staff nurse and those of nursing managers whose interests are opposed to her own:

Those people with their advanced degrees, the administrators, are no longer nurses. They're something else. They're administrators with different priorities. They can't relate to patient care anymore. All they can relate to is managing the institution, disciplining us and ordering supplies.

Understanding that staff and management nurses have opposing interests beyond common occupational concerns is insightful, considering management's persistent use of the traditional interpretation of professionalism as a coercive, anti-union tool. They barrage staff with "meritocratic individualist" hype that all nurses share the common trait of superiority over blue collar workers, given their greater credentialism and inherent merits. In presenting nursing as a monolithic occupation, they attempt to win staff nurses' allegiance to the occupation, away from their class alliances.

Goldblum's class identity, as reflected in her reinterpretation of professionalism and her distinction between the class position of staff and administrative nurses, was unequivocally connected to her experience in the workplace. Like Halle's "workingmen" who differentiate between productive (blue collar) and nonproductive (white collar) workers (Halle, 1984), Heather Goldblum distinguished between administrators (mental workers) and nurses (manual patient care workers), the latter of whom "do work." Unlike Halle's workingmen, however, Heather Goldblum's class identity, along with that of many other frontline nurses, is based solely on her position at work, not by her position outside work (Halle, 1984; Halle and Romo, 1991).

The volley over the years between Goldblum's nonwork identity, as the college-educated wife of a physician, her factory-like work experience as a staff nurse, and the traditional ideology of professionalism as imposed by management, led her to reshape the ideology of professionalism into a concept that connotes greater latitude over personal decision making at work. This is the process Wilentz described concerning the formation of class-based ideologies, where "old ideas are rearticulated into different class perceptions." Goldblum's class position at work transformed her interpretation of professionalism. Although the traditional interpretation is omnipresent, in memos from administration, in hospital committee meetings, in nursing journals and schools, and in daily conversation, nurses imbue it with meaning that corresponds to their own work experience.

The work experience of most nurses in a low class position leads them to reject meritocratic individualism as embodied in the managerial use of professionalism. They came to discover that this form of administrative control is simply a smokescreen, intended to cloud the divergent class interests within the occupation. Nurses in this class position see that it fails to assuage their problems at work.

Brenda Murphy, the head nurse in the gynecology clinic at Mt. Zion Hospital, bluntly rejected this form of managerial control. She came to work at Mt. Zion 15 years ago—accidently, she says. She liked it, graduated from a three-year nursing school with a diploma, and has stayed ever since. She has always considered nursing a hobby, not a career, because she too enjoys the altruism of patient care. She feels that nursing is caught up in an "identity crisis," however, and is trapped and mangled by "professionalism." While other more autonomous occupations have absorbed women into their professional ranks (often onto the lowest rungs), nursing has been left behind as a subordinate, low-paid, pink collar ghetto. To allay their insecurity, some nurses (from all class positions) latch onto the traditional, individualist interpretation of professionalism, which they want to believe will miraculously imbue them with social and economic mobility. Others, like Brenda Murphy, "have seen the light" and believe organizing for collective control over work conditions, rather than pursuit of capitalist individualist principles (e.g., market control for profit maximization), will bear the fruits of their labor and bring "true professionalism":

I find the meaning of professionalism [they impose on us] a crock of shit. The whole term makes me sick. You do what you do, and you do it well. That's all. If you need more staff or resources to do your work (caring for patients), demand it! Organize, have a "sickout," do whatever it takes.

Being able to give better care—that's being a professional.

Other staff nurses adamantly support Murphy's view. Betty Jean Alario, a staff nurse who has worked in St. John's ICU for the past nine years, bitterly described the way in which management abuses the concept of professionalism to increase the workload and culpability of staff nurses. Alario was the Mother Jones of St. John's Hospital. I met her at the side entrance of the hospital, and we walked together through a maze of hidden passageways that only an employee would know how to follow. On our way to the cafeteria, people stopped her to tell her about problems on their own units, on their friends' floors, and to kibitz with her. It was clear that Alario, college educated, strong and confident in her views, originally "laid back" (as she described herself), was a central figure in collective organizing at the hospital. She had developed a clear sense of the way in which management used professionalism to manipulate nurses, imposing a commandment of "service before thyself," with nothing in return. In spite of this coercion, Betty Jean Alario still strives for the work control interpretation of professionalism to which she, and many of her colleagues in a low class position, subscribe: self-determination in the workplace as a reward for their altruistic service, hard work, and expertise. She speaks candidly:

I realized I was not considered a professional. The hospital uses professionalism for their own means: you shouldn't organize, you're here to help the sick and should do so. . . . But then you turn around, and they're rotating shifts on you. Or you're understaffed; you need a medication and you go to pharmacy to get it. Something may happen and the hospital says to you, "You're responsible. You shouldn't have left the bedside. You're a professional."

They use this professionalism thing. They lay off aides and LPNs and then say to us, "Why don't you clean up the sink? Don't you think its professional to make it nice for our clients?" Or they say, "Pick up the garbage; it's unprofessional to leave it there." We get all the work and they say to us that a professional would do it for the patient, because they're committed to helping the sick.

To me, a professional is someone who excels in work, has autonomy . . . it could be anyone. A housekeeper could be a professional.

Alario's work experience, with staff shortages, rotating shifts, and extra housekeeping duties, clarified the way in which management uses professionalism to control nurses. To cut costs, they shrink the labor force and pile the excess work on staff nurses, informing them that balking is indicative of "unprofessional" behavior. Despite the transparency of this duplicitous managerial strategy, the broader cultural construct of the Protestant work ethic remains pervasive in the workplace. In return for their hard work and devotion to the greater good, nurses in a low class position feel morally deserving of reward. The reality that frontline nurses are denied such rewards, however, given their adherence to this cultural principle, leads to their own class-based politics, in the form of trade unionism, to rectify the conflict.

As these examples illustrate, the majority of nurses in a low class position (84 percent) reject the capitalist individualist interpretation of the ideology of professionalism as a selfish, undesirable goal and as an inaccurate portrayal of their experience in the workplace. They reinterpret the ideology into collective control over work, based on their class-based experience in the workplace. Lacking lunch and bathroom breaks, adequate personnel, and being forced to sign in and out easily defines their map of social reality. They perceive of themselves as workers, in opposition to a management that subjects them to factory-like rules. Pursuing their own class-based interpretation of professionalism leads nurses in a low class location to develop an autonomous politics of collectivism, of trade unionism.

Choice of Collective Strategy: Trade or Professional Unionism

In attempting to attain increased control over the conditions of their work, 98 percent of the nurses from a low class position spoke of some form of unionism as their most viable strategic alternative. The majority of those nurses, 60 percent, wanted trade unionism, 34 percent wanted professional unionism, and 6 percent wanted either trade or professional unionism. (See Appendix A, questions 17 and 18, in the survey instrument and Appendix B for coding of those questions.) Of these, 60 percent chose trade unionism as the means to enhance their control over the conditions of work, 20 percent wanted professional unionism for the same goal, and 4 percent wanted either trade or professional unionism for increased control over their work. Thus, 84 percent wanted some form of unionism to attain control over workplace issues. Eleven percent of the nurses in a low class position wanted professional unionism for both increased control and status, and 5 percent in the low class position wanted professional unionism for simply increased status. One nurse (2.3 percent) was unsure what she wanted.

If 60 percent of the nurses from a low class position in this study supported trade unionism as their form of collective strategy, why then did the professional union, the NYSNA, win the election at each institution? How does the historical-political context affect the expression of strategy? There are two central issues that must be addressed in order to evaluate the seeming contradiction between the actual vote for NYSNA at each hospital and nurses' (in a low class position) stated preference for trade unionism in this study: sophisticated anti-union management techniques and the political state of the trade union itself.[1]

Anti-Union Techniques

The techniques that hospital management use in their attempt to prevent trade unionism cannot be minimized. The workplace is, as, Richard Edwards (1979) wrote, a "contested terrain," where management and workers continually jockey for position. One technique management employs is something as simple as "auditing" their staff--keeping their finger on the pulse of workers' activities--to "head trade unionism off at the pass," as Sam McLaughlin, a middle manager from St. John's' Hospital, described it. McLaughlin was hired by St. John's Hospital only three and a half months prior to our interview but had been previously employed as a nursing supervisor for 30 years by a hospital in Lynn,

Massachusetts, which had brought in a consulting firm well known as a "union-busting outfit" according to McLaughlin.

A union-management committee met daily during union campaigns at this hospital in Massachusetts to exercise "corrective management," as the firm labeled it. McLaughlin took part in courses taught by these consultants, who advised nursing managers to spend more time "auditing" their staff, to find out personal details on nurses' concerns in order to "correct deficiencies" before the nurse decided to go to a union for help. McLaughlin was to determine which staff felt content, which dissatisfied, and which were leaders or followers. She was also instructed to intrude into the private lives of her staff and discern whether their problems were work related or love related (the only two alternatives offered). The consultants showed films explaining that unions use certain "inflammatory words," such as *workers* or *lack of respect* to trigger emotional reactions among staff. Management was instructed to steer clear of such language and instead use terms like *professional* and *sophisticated*. Administration was also advised to encourage a more cooperative management style, minimizing confrontation between management and staff.

McLaughlin, implementing these teachings, developed new channels of communication between staff and management, allowing staff to choose a representative from each floor, to carry the requests and complaints directly to the vice president of nursing who would "love to hear from them." This style of corrective management is a variation on participatory management, critiqued as another union-busting technique, whereby direct worker input to management is intended to circumvent the traditional need for worker representation (unions), theoretically eliminating the need for unions altogether.

Mt. Zion Hospital used similar techniques during the nurses' union campaign in 1982. The traditional anti-union strategy of "spying" on workers was employed as Mt. Zion administration audited nurses' every move, detailed in memos from nursing supervisors to the vice president (Archives, 1982). Hospital security was deployed by nursing administration to spy on staff nurses who were attempting to organize on the units (personal correspondence).

Frontline nurses at Mt. Zion were ultimately unsuccessful in their attempts to prevent management from spying on them, since the vice president was meticulous with her middle managers, ensuring that they scrupulously documented the staff activities. She requested feedback on all union activity on the units regarding "tempo and rumors, determination of the facts, and who is showing activity. . . . [They were told to] . . . obtain copies of any literature being circulated on the units." In addition, she directed her supervisors to monitor nurses' time and determine whether their sick days were actually being used for "in-house campaigning," and if so, put a halt to it.

The traditional ideology of professionalism was heavily employed by the nursing administration during the union campaign as well. The vice president directed her managers to challenge the professionalism, or purity of "white collaredness," among those staff nurses leaning toward trade unionism. In a memo to her managers, she wrote, "take a (subtle) position that there is a need for 'professionalism': staff nurses should be encouraged to select the representation that best suits their needs" (personal correspondence), thus using her position as a bully pulpit as well.

Nursing management played a leading role in shaping the outcome of the union election. First and foremost, they pushed for no union. Second, they implicitly endorsed NYSNA over either of the trade unions (the AFT or Local 1199) (personal correspondence). The vice president of nursing instructed the nursing staff to "maintain the highest standards of professional nursing practice," a seemingly innocent affirmation of professionalism by nursing management. However, this was also the slogan NYSNA used in its campaign as well, another of management's subtle attempts to undermine trade unionism.[2] Finally, the vice president implicitly encouraged nurses to vote "no union," since by mere coincidence, none of the trade unions appeared on the ballot distributed. These sorts of not-so-subtle tactics were, according to staff nurses, used repeatedly by the administration to counter union efforts.

Another tactic Mt. Zion management used, enabling the professional association to prevail, was recruitment of Filipino nurses (Archives, Medical Staff letter, March 1981). These nurses were afraid of losing their visas as well as their jobs, and therefore easily toed the managerial line. As Mt. Zion staff nurse Jenny Cornwell put it, "The biggest defeat of the union came from the foreign nurses. They're scared to death of management. They don't speak the language well, they're afraid of losing their visas, and they'll do anything they're told."

Federal labor law is another strategy skillfully used by hospital managements across the country to prevent unionism. In 1981, Presbyterian-St. Luke's Medical Center in Denver, Colorado, for example, won a suit that held that the NLRB must prevent proliferation of bargaining units in the health care industry. This decision had the effect of preventing unionization because it meant hospitals could increase the size of their bargaining units, which decreased the number of units before a union campaign. This hurt union elections because the larger the size of the bargaining unit, the less the likelihood of unionism (Fink and Greenberg, 1989: 172).

These managerial techniques--using stool pigeons, distorting the facts, emphasizing elitism and differences among workers, bringing in scared, foreign laborers, challenging federal labor laws, and delaying elections for years--while not particularly unusual in the history of American labor, are still effective in countering the work control ideology that I found among 84 percent of the nurses in a low class position at Mt. Zion and St. John's hospitals. Management journals have in fact reported that hospitals have become "more skilled in resisting unionization efforts." In 1968 unions won about 83 percent of the hospital elections across the country, whereas by the mid-1970s it had fallen to 55 percent (Fink and Greenberg, 1989: 169) By 1986, over 20 percent of all RNs had collective bargaining agreements. Of those, 50 percent or 120,000, are represented by ANA state affiliates, and 60,000 by trade unions: 30,000 by Service Employees International Union, 20,000 by Local 1199, and about 10,000 by independent unions (Brint, 1986: 50).

Internal Union Politics: The League of Registered Nurses, 1199

The politics of the particular union in question also played a crucial role in influencing nurses' choice of collective strategy to attain their vision of professionalism. The nurses at St. John's Hospital had been members of the League of Registered Nurses, Local 1199, along with nurses' aides, LPNS, orderlies, and other auxiliary hospital workers since 1980. Ultimately they decided they had no choice but to decertify Local 1199 and join the professional union, NYSNA, as a result of the trade union's serious deterioration. The League of Registered Nurses division of Local 1199 was initially established in 1977 by Sondra Clarke, at Brookdale Medical Center, for nurses who were dissatisfied with the ANA and its complicity with management. By 1982, nurses in eight institutions in New York City, including St. John's Hospital, had decertified NYSNA for Local 1199..

St. John's nurses initially brought in Local 1199 because of the disarray in their work conditions: indiscriminate layoffs, lack of autonomy, health and safety problems, discrimination against minorities, and favoritism in promotions, merit raises, and suspensions. Robin Mintener, a head nurse at St. John's Hospital and one of the organizers of Local 1199 at the hospital, feels that eventually nurses gained confidence that the trade union was solidly behind them on these issues.

By 1984 their world had turned upside down. In July of that year, the Local 1199 Hospital and Guild Division's citywide contract with the League of Voluntary Hospitals had expired. Doris Turner, the new president of New York Local 1199, the hand-picked successor of Leon Davis who had started the union in 1934, was seeking a new contract that would include every other weekend off. The hospitals resisted the union's demand and offered only 26 weekends off. (Thus, the hospital could distribute weekends off all in a row rather than evenly throughout the year.) This issue became Turner's cause célébre, and on July 13, 1984, she ordered 50,000 union members at 41 institutions to participate in shutting down the city's hospitals.

Before the strike had even been called, St. John's' nurses had already lost patience with the new leadership at Local 1199. Sondra Clarke had resigned in 1983, under pressure from Turner, and St. John's nurses felt their relationship with the union was irretrievably slipping. Their grievances were not followed up, and at the monthly delegate assembly meetings, Doris Turner would intimidate and otherwise verbally abuse the nurses, publicly disclaiming them as elitist and challenging their very presence in the union. Nurses reported they were never recognized by Turner for the floor, and many stopped going to delegate assembly altogether, devising their own plan of action. They had a window period to decertify, 120 days before their own contract expired, and some nurses had negotiated a separate St. John's' benefit package for themselves. "There was a gigantic split among nurses about going with NYSNA," says Robin Mintener, although "they knew that [having] no union was absolutely suicidal."

The strike itself was totally disorganized. Nurses from St. John's Hospital sought information from the leadership on the strike, and it was never forthcoming. Of 400 nurses at St. John's, only 63 voted, and of those, only 38 voted to strike. Two hundred nurses finally did go on strike, but more out of confusion, fear, and support of nonnurses whose contract was on the line than out of commitment to the union. After the third day, only 80 stayed out. Of those, Mintener surmised, the majority struck purely out of sympathy with trade unionism itself, not with Local 1199 per se. "We felt the ideology of trade unionism was very important so we stuck together," she says. Nevertheless, relationships between nurses began breaking down. Some crossed the picket line and were inside the hospital decertifying the union, while others walked.

Betty Jean Alario, who chose to strike, explained that management took advantage of the mass confusion and began to intimidate the nurses. They called striking nurses into their offices one at a time and told them that court orders were out for them. Alario, as one of the union leaders, was held captive in management offices late into the night. When the nurses contacted the union on this matter for guidance and support, they were told, "It's every man for himself." After two weeks of striking, 12 nurses from St. John's Hospital went to the Roosevelt Hotel at 3 a.m. to talk to the union leadership. The nurses were shut out, unable to speak directly to Doris Turner, and were told to leave the premises or they would be arrested.

The strike was completely disorganized at the senior-most level of the union from the start. Turner never called her executive council together to agree to the terms of the strike. It was, as Fink and Greenberg describe it, "a test of wills between Turner and the hospitals" (Fink and Greenberg, 1989: 223). Although 80 percent of the membership already had every other weekend off, Turner pursued a 10 percent wage increase and every other weekend off. Picket signs were never made, picket lines were small, and a requisite 10-day filing notice by nurses at St. John's and three other hospitals was overlooked (resulting in $600,000 worth of fines to the union). The union is legally obligated to give the hospital 10 days' notice before a strike; Local 1199 told the nurses it had provided notice, but it had not.

These problems, along with the frustrations that preceded the strike, prompted nurses at four institutions, including St. John's, to decertify. The issue, however, was less about the ideology of trade unionism than it was about the nurses' pragmatic need for strong representation in the workplace. The union was a collapsing house of cards, and everyone knew it. As Betty Jean Alario put it, "We pragmatic need for strong representation in the workplace. The union was a collapsing house of cards, and everyone knew it. As Betty Jean Alario put it, "We believed in collective bargaining and in 1199. The problem was just that 1199 wasn't representing nurses properly. We felt our only other option at the time was NYSNA."

Trade Unionism Versus Professional Unionism: The Straighter Path to Work Control Professionalism

Despite the collapse of the trade union and union-busting techniques, 60 percent of the nurses interviewed, in a low class position from St. John's and Mt. Zion hospitals, still supported trade unionism as the strongest vehicle for attaining their vision of professionalism. (This is a remarkable figure given that national union membership hovers at approximately 17 percent.) These nurses felt that the professional union, an arm of the professional association, NYSNA, was unacceptable. It reproduced the major elements of the traditional ideology of professionalism, which they found reprehensible. The professional union was both unwilling and unable to address their interests at work. These nurses emphasized the need for a "real" union--a trade union with experience, clout, and interests in its members' needs.

Nurses in a low class position saw NYSNA as embracing the meritocratic individualist incarnation of professionalism, because its primary motive is to promote the prestige of the occupation, not workplace demands. These nurses described NYSNA as solely committed to controlling the entry gates to nursing by elevating the educational degree requirements and the class background of nursing practitioners. This NYSNA goal is clearly evident in its endorsement of ANA's Entry into Practice position: relegate staff nursing as it is currently practiced (involved with patient contact) to a low-status manual job, and elevate supervisory nursing as it is currently practiced (coordinating the tasks of other care givers) to a high-status, "mental" career, requiring credentialism.

Brenda Murphy, head nurse from the gynecology clinic at Mt. Zion who rejected the individualist ideology of professionalism, also rejects this NYSNA angle on the transformation of nursing. She believes the association is actually destroying the essence of nursing, contact with patients, while promoting the "mental," white collar, paper-pushing activities, over and above the often dirty, manual labor required in bedside care. In so doing, nurses are denied satisfaction in work, helping others, as they are forced to focus on theory or management rather than patients:

NYSNA are a bunch of old biddies. I never liked them as a union or as a professional association. They disrupted nursing. It used to be a hands-on profession. By requiring a B.S.N., nurses don't get experience in the hospital anymore, and they have *no* concept

TEXAS STATE TECH. COLLEGE
LIBRARY-SWEETWATER TX.

of patients . . . who are up to their necks in shit.

NYSNA calls confronting patient care as experiencing culture shock. They don't want to take care of patients. . . . They don't want to dirty their little hands. Prestige is what's important to them.

Jenny Cornwell corroborates Murphy's perceptions on the erosion of nursing. She believes NYSNA has denigrated frontline nursing work, to pave the way for its pursuit of power, prestige, and credentialism:

NYSNA has fostered this idea that the very worst thing a bright, educated female could do is become a staff nurse. They don't like practicing nursing. All they're interested in is getting more letters [degrees] after their names.

Others are angry with the way in which NYSNA equates credentialism with professionalism. NYSNA has been lobbying for the 1985 proposal, a proposal to change the educational degree requirements for entry into nursing. This proposal would require all RNs to have college degrees (a B.S.N.) by 1985, a date that has been extended to 1995. Those without such a degree would ostensibly be relegated to the subordinate position of technical nurse.

Joanie Williams, whom I visited in her Mt. Zion-owned apartment on the edge of Harlem, along with many others, sees nothing inherently wrong with more education for nurses. (In fact, many embrace education as a means for becoming better practitioners.) What they object to is the college degree requirement for RN licensure, which they predict would solidify the stratification in nursing according to both class background and education. Only those able to afford a four-year college education would become an RN; those unable would remain the lesser "technical" nurses, cementing inequality within nursing, which they believe is NYSNA's ulterior motive. If it were not, Williams suggests, the professional association would force hospitals to reimburse all nurses for their education, as trade unions have done for their members:

When I was an aide, in 1199, the hospital paid for my way to go to school. . . . That 1985 proposal, though, I hate that proposal. Those "ladies" [the educators and administrators] in NYSNA, the standards-setting body, should have facilitated education for all of us, for everyone. They're always kickin' and screamin' about education . . . but they already have theirs.

So why don't they force management to give us tuition reimbursement like the union does? It's obvious "1985" is just for themselves. The rest, about more education for nurses, is just a lot of bull.

Such nurses in a low class position clearly reject the individualist conception of professionalism as promoted by NYSNA: individual and occupational prestige and power achieved via credentialism. They also reject NYSNA for pretending to be what it is not--a "real" union.

Staff nurses at Mt. Zion descried the unfair relationship nursing administration holds with NYSNA, placing frontline nurses between a rock and a hard place. Mt. Zion nursing administrators also sit on the board of directors of the professional association. These same administrators vote on labor issues that come before the General and Economic Welfare Committee of NYSNA while simultaneously sitting on the side of management during contract negotiations with NYSNA. This blatant conflict of interest had stoked the fires for decertification of the professional union at Mt. Zion.

Ellen Precht summed up this overt affront to Mt. Zion staff nurses. She is a staff nurse with two small children and has been actively involved in developing an on-site day care center for hospital employees. Her husband, who is a lawyer, has acted as the informal counsel for Mt. Zion nurses engaged in the decertification efforts. She describes the problem with NYSNA in this way:

NYSNA is not set up to be a good labor organization. It is a professional organization where any nurse can be a member. Nursing administrators from this hospital are on NYSNA's board of directors. NYSNA has their annual convention, and anyone can attend; any issue can come up, like how much money should go to General and Economic Welfare. Nursing administrators and educators from [Mt. Zion] *should not be voting on these issues*! It's just not right.

Other nurses sat talking with me in a nearby bakery for hours one Saturday afternoon, condemning NYSNA for perpetrating such a conflict of interest and for disguising itself as a union. Having lost the attempt to decertify the professional union, Jenny Cornwell was at her wit's end. She described the administrators' actions as a "farce" but felt she could no longer fight them. She "could participate in only one revolution in her lifetime," and her involvement in the attempt to oust NYSNA was it. Nevertheless, she was unwavering in her support of trade unionism over the professional union:

I feel positive about trade unions because as a union, their job is to run a union. They are not nurses disguised as union people, like NYSNA. Also, with a trade union you don't have management nurses on both sides of the bargaining table. Here, nursing managers sit on the opposite side of the table from me and vote on general and economic welfare issues *with* me. It's a joke. It's an obvious conflict of interest.

Initially, the biggest thing I had against NYSNA was their grievance procedures and negotiations. It was just a series of ineptitudes [*sic*]. But when we complained to the higher-ups, it became clear to us that it wasn't just a problem of inexperienced reps. NYSNA wasn't the least bit interested in staff patient ratios, *our* issues.

Not only were these frontline nurses outraged that NYSNA was a wolf in sheep's clothing, but many rejected the professional union for its values and goals--its focus on promotion of occupational status rather than workplace issues. As Nancy Hughley, a Mt. Zion staff nurse, put it, they wanted an organization to fight for and protect their interests at work, not to lie in bed with management:

NYSNA says they are and they aren't a union. Well, they don't represent nurses. . . . They're not interested in our needs. . . . I'm tellin' you, no one cheered louder than management when NYSNA won around here. They're all in it together. NYSNA gets our money, and the hospital gets power.

These nurses were angry with the actual influence NYSNA had over other nurses. By promoting the coercive, managerial aspects of professionalism--that nurses are too elite to walk a picket line--NYSNA contributed to their powerlessness. Nurses are, in Nancy Hughley's words, imprisoned by "the golden handcuff syndrome": seduced by false flattery and real perquisites they cannot afford to do without:

Most nurses feel powerless. They get these grandiose ideas about themselves in nursing school, from NYSNA, that they're professionals, an elite, and they shouldn't walk a picket line. So a lot of 'em accept this bullshit. On top of that, the hospital with NYSNA get you with the "golden handcuff syndrome." They give you perks that make you a prisoner. To leave my job I'd have to leave my apartment, and you know what that means in a place like New York!

Many nurses, having been previously caught in the web of professionalism as woven by NYSNA, sought to avoid it after they worked the hospital floors for a few years. They learned that NYSNA's promotion of meritocratic individualism via the doctrine of professionalism does not coincide with their own experience, and they seek "real unions" instead.

Laura Buddai, a head nurse in the ambulatory care clinic, originally from a small town in Trinidad, described how NYSNA seduces and disorients its members. She has worked at Mt. Zion Hospital for 13 years and currently moonlights with the U.S. Army Reserves, providing her with an annual salary of $35,000. Calling herself working class, nevertheless, she explained how the professional association jumbles reality:

I guess NYSNA tried to brainwash us all along. They always said, "You're professionals so you should stay with NYSNA; it's the only organization for professional nurses. Only nurses can know about nursing." Well, I finally said I don't care *who* represents me as long as they give good benefits and *really* represent us.

Ideological Formation

Several nurses in the low class position lent insight into how they came to reject the "brainwashing" of NYSNA, similar to the process Wilentz described as ideological formation: confrontation, negotiation, and redefinition (Wilentz, 1983). Nurses' problematic social realities forced confrontation with the individualist interpretation of professionalism foisted on them from above. As they redefined professionalism to meet their own understanding of their workplace experience, it coalesced into a politics of trade unionism for many staff nurses.

Betty Jean Alario, who had worked as a staff nurse at St. John's for nine years, described her personal transformation, from "an elitist nurse" unwilling to associate with blue collar trade unions (which she initially saw as violent and corrupt), into a professional health care "worker," sharing common problems and needs with other health care workers. Her experience with arbitrary promotions and firings, disregard for occupational health hazards, and inadequate compensation jolted her into becoming a strong trade union supporter. She felt she could no longer afford her false sense of security as socially superior to others:

When 1199 first came around, I was extremely anti-union, elitist. . . . In no way should a professional be in a union. . . . They are for blue collar workers only.

I used to be so laid back. But, I tell you, I couldn't *help* getting involved. The issue around here wasn't economics. It was things like merit raises determined by personality or being fired at the whim of your supervisor. Or, if you used your own judgment on something, they could get rid of you. There were also a lot of other unfair labor practices, like no safety for nurses. For example, we were using this liniment, DMSO, on cancer patients, which we thought would have toxic fumes. A lot of pregnant nurses were using this stuff, and we were worried.

Well, finally I started going to union meetings, and the more I went the more I learned. That I am a worker and I should have certain rights. As a worker, you're entitled to pay, compensation, safety on the job. . . . I finally agreed that as a health care worker we should go with 1199 because it dealt with all health care workers. . . . We were all involved with health care, and we should be there to support each other.

Other nurses from St. John's portrayed similar processes of ideological transformation, from meritocratic individualist to cooperative collectivist, influenced by their rude awakenings at work. Although the individualist interpretation of professionalism, taught in nursing schools and on the hospital floors, is a powerful motivator, it is not powerful enough to arrest the change nurses go through from their workplace experiences. Fiona Edelman, a staff nurse who has worked at St. John's for 15 years, explained how mistreatment of other workers was a much more forceful educator than managerial rhetoric on professionalism. She saw colleagues who had worked at the hospital for decades being dropped like flies. She figured somewhere down the line it might be her. Fear for her own job overrode whatever traces were left from her elitist sense of self, and she started to feel that trade unions were the only viable challenge to management's authority:

I'm not very political. I lead a very busy life. But I think management is trying to make life uncomfortable for nurses. An older nurse had made an error, and, after 20 years here, they fired her, just like that. Twenty years. That could easily be me.

We were taught in nursing school in your first intro course, "The Fundamentals of Nursing," that nurses are professionals and don't join unions. They tell you this all through school, along with other basics like how to give a bed bath or take vital signs.

But I've seen unions help people. They get you good benefits and give you more job security. I saw that if the administration did something to you, someone is there working for you, to protect you. Administrators are afraid of unions; it's a challenge to their authority. We need that here. My mother always told me unions are good, unions are good; and now I agree with her. What they told us in school just doesn't make sense.

Even Joanie Williams, who stood up to her supervisors by calling her union representative when they tried to corner her for arriving late, initially bought into the rhetoric that unions are evil and vile:

I used to believe unions just wanted to get money from workers and be violent—slashin' tires and what-not during strikes. But I saw they did a lot for the workers. They get money for their members and protect you from your supervisors if they harass you.

Williams changed her tune over the course of her 16 years at Mt. Zion Hospital. Managerial intimidation taught her that the culture of meritocracy cannot protect her job. After arriving late one morning, her supervisor cornered her, trying to cower her into submission. Williams described it thusly:

She tried to get her gang against me. . . . Two supervisors, one coordinator and you [me]. They put you on the hot seat. . . . Most people give in, but not me, Joanie Williams.

I said, "I'm calling my delegate *now*. You want to meet with me, then you are going to have to meet with me *and* my delegate." Suddenly her voice changed, and she said, "Now I don't see why we have to make a big thing about all this. I just want to talk to you."

I knew she wanted to intimidate me with her gang. But I knew my rights as a union member. They expect you to shut up and take it. With my delegate there, . . . it did not go into my folder.

During her years in the hospital, Williams came to see herself as a "light blue collar worker" in need of a strong trade union to protect her interests on the job. Crosscutting occupations and creating her own blue collar-white collar color lines, Williams zeroed in on class position, arguing that all nonmanagerial employees need representation by trade unions:

Trade unions should only be for blue collar workers. White collar workers don't need 'em. Now it depends what you're callin' a white collar worker. I think they're the supervisors and executive types. I don't consider myself one of them. At $35,000 I'm a light blue collar worker. Anyone earning less than $40,000[3] is a blue collar worker. You say some assistant professors earn $28,000? I'd say they're deep deep blue collar; in bad need of a union.

Williams's belief in the need for trade unionism was in concert with her work control interpretation of professionalism. Trade unions are a means to gain greater control over the conditions of work. Individual and occupational prestige through monopoly control over the nursing market, the capitalist individualist interpretation of professionalism, does not enter into her equation.

It can be concluded that most (60 percent) nurses who see themselves as workers react politically in accordance with the class identity they have formed: they adopt trade unionism. They perceive it as the only viable strategy to facilitate arriving at their vision of professionalism: greater self-determination at work and improved bread-and-butter rewards, in recognition of their hard work, skill, and devotion to their patients. Their class identity, perception of themselves as workers in conflict with management that deprives them of what they see as rightfully theirs (self-determination, adequate salaries, staff, and dignity at work), surfaced and solidified during their experience in the workplace. Understanding their vision of professionalism as an ideology of work control provided a window through which I was able to peruse class identity in formation.

Most rejected professional unionism because it perpetuated management's interests, not their own. Hence, the autonomous politics that emerged from the development of frontline nurses' worldview was trade unionism. A minority of nurses in a low class position supported professional unionism--34 percent. Of those, 20 percent did so as a vehicle to attain control over the conditions of their work, and 11 percent did so to achieve both status and work control.

It must be remembered, however, that hospitals are contested terrains. This means nurses' choice of collective strategy is often muddied by such issues as sophisticated anti-union techniques employed by hospital management and the internal politics of particular trade unions. In order to understand why these nurses would support a collective bargaining representative whose goals are antithetical to their own, one must seriously consider the role of these other powerful factors.

MEDIUM CLASS POSITION

Nurses in the medium class position, like those in a low class position, also wanted to view themselves as professionals, but they infused professionalism with meaning that is more inclusive than collective control over work conditions. For 76 percent of the nurses in a medium class position, professionalism signifies a composite of both work control and popular individualism (a perception that their personal freedom from unwelcome economic, ideological, and political constraints will emerge from compliant behaviors and credentialism). This form of professionalism incorporates the individualist culture of meritocracy into its worldview. Individual credentialism and compromising behaviors are perceived as the solution to their collective problems at work. Although 24 percent of these nurses define professionalism as work control, the majority in this class position are more heavily wrapped in the American cultural traditions of individualism.

Diana Marcos is a middle managerial nurse originally from the Philippines who has worked at Mt. Zion for the past eight and a half years. For her, professionalism means having increased authority over her work (more autonomy over patient care and input into hospital policies) and a more refined white collar image: a baccalaureate degree and proper dress, speech, and attitudes at work. These characteristics, Marcos believes, should ensure her individual access to the American dream.

When Diana Marcos and her husband, a chemist, arrived in this country, they started a business in Westchester County with a few of their relatives, selling imported rattan furniture from the Philippines. Soon after both found employment in their respective fields. During her early years at Mt. Zion, Marcos was intimidated and withdrawn from most activities. Like other Filipino nurses, she was insecure about losing her visa. Subsequently she became an active member of various nursing committees, especially those promoting a white collar persona for nurses. She became, for example, a member of the Professional Image Committee, which tries to foster a more middle-class image for nurses, with "polished attitudes, dress and speech." She is the leader of a Bi-cultural Nursing Program, which instructs non-U.S.-born nursing graduates to maintain a "professional" (nonantagonistic) demeanor in the face of inevitable conflict on the units with patients, physicians, and management. Despite these efforts to project a more mainstream, white collar picture of nursing, Diana Marcos is still concerned with her relative impotence as a nurse when it comes to control over her own work conditions. Her vision of professionalism reflects these mixed concerns with her work and individual status:

Professionalism is having more say about what happens to us at this hospital as far as work conditions, input on hospital policies, rules, and regulations and how we care for our patients. . . . Unfortunately, we have very little of this.

Society pays for what they think is professional. So, I'm on the "professional image committee," trying to change the image of nursing--make it more professional. We're trying to upgrade nursing by requiring a B.S.N. degree, polishing nurses' attitudes, their dress, the way they speak, their general demeanor.

The reinterpretation of the ideology of professionalism by nurses in a medium class position reflects the more contradictory nature of their class location: they are simultaneously managers and employees. As a result of their employee status, nurses in the medium class position are interested in gaining more authority over the conditions of their work. But their partial managerial status leads them in pursuit of individualistic goals: increasing their prestige and power (their personal freedom) through the human capital strategy of credentialism.

Vaughn White, a middle manager at St. John's Hospital who occupies one of the recently created middle-level administrative nursing care coordinator positions, perceives professionalism in the same light as Marcos. Like most of these other mid-level nurses at St. John's, White was hired within the last four years from outside the hospital, with a master's degree. Management's intent was to increase the educational gap between staff and managerial nurses, to prevent alliances between them. White was previously employed for 11 years as a staff nurse in a hospital on Long Island but now characterizes herself, and her insurance salesman husband, as upwardly mobile "yuppies" who have not quite made it but are almost there, given their recent purchase of a home in Queens. Fresh from the master's in nursing mills, White exudes confidence that doctors really listen to her now, unlike before she received her degree:

When I tell physicians that this is the way it is (professional nurses have autonomy and . . . knowledge), they listen to me now. They recognize my clinical expertise.

A lot of nurses complain they have too much work to do. They should attend seminars and keep up to date. It's unprofessional to see it just as a job.

For nurses in a medium class position, the deeply ingrained meritocratic individualist message that power and prestige will come with credentialism takes precedence in their vision of professionalism. They believe they will be unable to get ahead in life if they cooperate or associate with lower-status blue collar workers (and their collective strategies) in their quest for greater authority in the workplace. The issue of work control therefore pales in comparison to their almost blind pursuit of power and prestige (their vision of personal freedom). In addition, a major component of their job as middle managers is to disseminate the administration's official line on professionalism to their subordinates. This official line, just like Mt. Zion's anti-union offensive, ascribes an individualist, noncollectivist approach to problems in the workplace. It focuses on individual social mobility as linked to improvement in human capital through credentialism and compliance with the goals of management.[4] Collective battles against management would, according to this view, result in degradation of status and power.

Silvie Hammond, another middle managerial nurse from St. John's, exemplifies this interpretation of professionalism. She, like most of the others, was hired by St. John's three and a half years earlier as a nursing care coordinator. Raised in the Bronx, where she worked as a staff nurse for 10 years prior to getting her master's in nursing and her position at St. John's, Hammond explained this blame-the-victim approach to nurses' problems:

Nurses who *feel* subservient to doctors, even if they think he's wrong, do what he tells them anyway. Nurses have to *feel* and *act* more autonomous. One way to feel better about yourself is to get more education.

In this unit we have problems with the doctor-nurse relationship. If a patient is deteriorating and a nurse wants to order a drug, the intern who just graduated from medical school has his ego on the line. He says, "No nurse is gonna tell me what to do."

Hammond offers the official line that despite the inequality between physicians and nurses, the latter can overcome that disparity through attitude changes and credentialism. This "self-esteem," human capital approach to changing power relations negates the material basis for the inequalities. That management controls the processes of economic, ideological, and political production in the hospital bureaucracy and that most physicians are still independent entrepreneurs controlling the processes of medical production are not factored into this analysis of change. Nurses, while levying gradations of control in the institution, are still its employees, regardless of their credentials, rendering them ultimately subordinate to management and physicians. Thus, the popular individualist view of professionalism, drawing on the culture of meritocracy, while espoused and internalized by mid-level nurses, becomes a device for managerial control over middle management, as well as over frontline nurses.

In an effort to enhance managerial control over nurses, nursing management has fought for another variant on professionalism: holding individual nurses legally liable for their actions, removing the onus from the hospital or supervisor. If this strategy were to succeed, it would force nurses within and between class positions to become even more divided in their interests. To avoid individual blame, they would be compelled to look out for their personal interests first and foremost, above and beyond any collective interests. Driving another wedge between individual nurses is another of management's attempts at preventing unionization. The more divided that staff are, the less likely it is that they will strive for collective solutions to what may seem like individual problems.

Charlotte Ramsey, the vice president of nursing at St. John's, explained that she is trying to impose such a view of professionalism on both her middle managers and staff nurses; success, she claims, would lead to increased staff productivity as well as higher profitability of the hospital as a whole:

We are trying to reeducate our nurses about "professional nursing," to be autonomous, accountable, and responsible. . . . By being intelligent, educated, hard working, accountable, responsible, and autonomous professionals, they'll be able to make business more profitable.

Her focus is once again on the individual nurse, away from the structural problems of the organization. Her primary interest is in transforming nursing workers, not nursing work. By equating professionalism with individual behaviors, the burden of responsibility for structural problems in the workplace (such as inadequate staff and supplies due to cost cutting) is transferred away from management to the individual. Clearly the roots of this blame-the-victim aspect of the professional are located in the cultural premises of meritocracy, whereby individuals are accorded personal responsibility for their own rise and fall due to their inherent strengths and weaknesses (Newman, 1988).

The individualist interpretation of professionalism takes precedence in the middle managers' composite vision of the ideology, which presents a serious conflict of interest for the very nurses who espouse this view. On the one hand, they do share in some of the status that the individualist interpretation memorializes, simply by virtue of their being members of management (on an admittedly low level). They meet with nursing management, have access to conference funds, are privy to certain types of managerial information, and have better salaries than staff nurses, yet their work conditions still reflect their subordination. They are subject to the authority of an array of nursing, medical, and administrative superiors who have another agenda: increasing the productivity and profitability of the hospital.

Seena Rocco, who has worked her way up from a junior college associate degree to a master's in nursing, embodies the ideological conflict of being both management and employee simultaneously. She is currently employed in St. John's renal and detoxification unit, where she has been since she was hired three years ago. She and her husband were born and raised on Staten Island where he is a certified public accountant. Together they earn a comfortable income. Yet Seena Rocco remains discontent with the conditions of her work. The work overload and sense of drudgery and servitude she experiences, even as a middle management nurse, overwhelm her:

Professionalism means having a degree and autonomy--taking responsibility for your care and not referring your problems to someone else.

But we still need more money, more prestige, and more power. You'd think if you had "expert power," you know, intelligence or degrees, you'd think you could go from there. But no. The average nurse doesn't go any further. Doctors, dentists . . . they don't have to push like we do to get anywhere.

You really have to slave in this profession. Fifty percent of the time is stressful. You can never do your work fast enough. We have to run to cardiac arrests; you stick yourself with needles all the time, slip on the waxed floors, lift heavy patients.

We have to be "*nice*" people all the time. We aren't supposed to care about how much money we make. We're only supposed to care about our patients.

When I went to school, I thought I'd be a nurse or maybe a teacher. I never thought it'd be like this.

Rocco's contradictory class interests lead her down a dead-end road. Her managerial interests lead her to seek greater personal freedom by improving her human capital, yet her interests as an employee lead her to seek changes in the conditions of her work--changes she cannot bring about. It is very difficult to alter the state of one's workplace conditions while shouldering full responsibility for them. Rocco's contradictory class interests cancel each other out.

Nevertheless, her individualist pursuit of power and prestige to rectify the economic, ideological, and political constraints on her in the workplace ultimately takes over. When asked whether she would ever change careers, her conflicted reply was, "No, I love my work. And anyway, there are lots of power positions still available in nursing" (her individualist solution to the collective problems facing mid-level nurses).

Despite internalizing and promoting upper management's official line on professionalism, nurses in a medium class position felt a great sense of frustration in not being able to attain their mixed vision. They remain unable to realize both the prestige and autonomy they are seeking. They smell the aroma of individual success as it is embodied by the physicians in their presence yet, cannot sink their teeth into it. They are taunted by the possibility of true power, prestige, and control in the workplace, but their contradictory class location yields no clear path to their goals.

The map of social reality constructed by nurses in the medium class position leads them to be at once captives and perpetrators of the individualist interpretation of professionalism. They are captives in that they are unsuccessfully pursuing the individualist, human capital road to salvation. They are perpetrators in that they willingly carry out a blame-the-victim form of managerial control, which contributes to the subordination of themselves, along with that of the frontline nurses.

This conflict is described by Mary Ellen Fein, a clinical supervisor in adult medicine at Mt. Zion. Although she tried to shoulder the responsibility for her problems at work by increasing her credentialism with a master's degree and promoted this approach with her staff, she still finds workplace problems beyond her grasp. The degree helped her gain some status in the eyes of other nurses, and with her fiancée's crowd of health care lawyers. It also helped her land the supervisory position she currently holds, but it has not given her the authority she needs to alter her work conditions. She experienced heavy burnout, since on top of her supervisory job, she finds herself being forced, along with staff nurses, to pick up duties that laid-off housekeepers, transporters, and technicians have left behind in the era of cost containment. She expresses exasperation with her role as perpetrator yet prisoner of professionalism:

You're really torn in two different directions. On the one hand you're trying to be professional: be responsible, assume accountability for your own practice--and instill the same ideas in the people you supervise.

But on the other hand, as nurses, we have to do whatever your supervisor assigns you, "for the needs of the patient." I didn't go to school to mop up the floor, to do the menial tasks that others were hired to do.

The frustration that Mary Ellen Fein describes illustrates the contradictory nature of the composite view on professionalism. While the human capital route enhanced her status somewhat, it did not imbue her with the power she needed to make changes in her work. In addition, management's use of professionalism as a coercive tool in the workplace became clearer to her as she too became caught in its clutches. Like many nurses in the low class position, she discovered that it can be used to impose more work on nurses as the need arises. She puts it succinctly:

Professionalism is a catchall phrase, like the Girl Scout's code of honor. Whatever your supervisor assigns you is what is professional.

Despite increasing frustration with their own ineffectiveness in maintaining control over their work, most middle management nurses do not forge alliances with lower-ranking employees, who are also seeking control over their work conditions. The pull from management is too strong. They focus on pushing harder for change within themselves and their occupation, an approach that does not threaten their meager hold on status. Their concern for regulating their conditions of work (greater autonomy, input into hospital policy, job safety, and fewer nonnursing tasks) is transformed into a concern with power in the hospital hierarchy. Hence, they advocate greater separation from blue collar strategies of resistance, and some go so far as to advocate the high-status, white collar strategies initiated by physicians pursued in the late 19th-century (which nurses in the high class location pursue wholeheartedly).

One middle management nurse supports medicine's individualist fee-for-service model as the solution to nurses' collective mistreatment. Debra Curry suffered a major bout of insecurity when her position as head nurse was eliminated at St. John's to remove it from the union, as rumor had it. She was then rehired as a "nursing care coordinator." Such reshuffling after 17 years of service jolted her into the realization that she is relatively powerless, even in her new middle managerial position. She first chose the human capital approach to solve these problems, getting her bachelor's degree, then her master's, to improve her own situation at the hospital. But it did not work. Rather than pursuing the collectivist strategy of unionism, from which she was removed, she advocates the only other alternative she found available: monopoly control over nursing.

Professionalism is having clout to make legislative changes for nursing in Washington and Albany—like getting ourselves fee for service the way physicians do. Nurses need to get paid for their teaching services.

I'm burnt out. I can never leave the floors even for a lunch break. I never have enough staff. . . . We can't focus on patient care anymore. Priorities are different now. Priorities are on paperwork, reports, nonnursing functions, statistics, and meetings. . . . If there's a problem, instead of solving it, they set up a meeting.

These middle management nurses remain stymied by their continued inability to break the barriers of the bureaucracy. They cannot repair its structural inequality, nor can they exert greater authority over their own domain. Adherence to the principles of popular individualism, pursuit of credentialism and compromise, as the road to personal salvation, led them into the magician's false trap door. They increased their personal worth with credentialism yet remain unable to exert self-determination in their work, despite some legislative change in the occupation. They remain subordinate employees.

Nurses in the medium class position, like those in the low class position, express their class identity through their interpretation of professionalism. But it is a conflicted identity, reflecting their conflicted membership in both management, ensconced in "meritocratic individualism," and downtrodden workers, although management has the greater pull.

Located as they are in this contradictory class position, 76 percent of the middle management nurses strive for a conflicted interpretation of professionalism: both work control (increased autonomy, job security, and input into hospital policies and fewer nonnursing tasks) and popular individualism (credentialism and compliant behavior). However, as they are pulled more toward their managerial than their employee position, they are unable to let go of their dogged pursuit of prestige. Hence, they are drawn more toward the individualist interpretation of professionalism to achieve their composite portrait. Their focus is thus directed toward changing the characteristics of themselves, their subordinates, and their occupation, not workplace conditions.

Trade Unionism or Professional Unionism: The Straighter Path to Power, Prestige, and Control at Work

Professional unionism is in concert with this composite vision of professionalism because it focuses on exalting nursing prestige and power in the workplace (which unionists often refer to as nursing practice issues). Its primary objective is to promote "proper behavior" and educational credentialism to attain these ends. Professional unions do employ collective bargaining, yet rather than adopt an antagonistic relationship toward management, as trade unions generally do, they attempt compromise with management at all cost. Ninety-four percent of the nurses in the medium class position support professional unionism.

Most middle managers advocate "working things out" with management rather than "blowing things out of proportion," and filing grievances, which trade unions might do. Debra Curry articulates this compromise position clearly. Ironically, she also describes herself as a member of the working class since she "has to work to live," as she puts it. Being a divorced, single mother, with a daughter in college and a son about to enter, she says she cannot afford to quit. She defines her support of professional unionism like this:

Unlike 1199 [the trade union that St. John's nurses recently decertified], NYSNA would understand that everything doesn't have to go to arbitration or grievance. NYSNA would try to work things out with management first.

If a unit were dangerously understaffed, the trade union would probably blow it all out of proportion and have it written up. NYSNA would try to work it out with administration. They'd probably hire an agency nurse to work the floor instead of grieving it. They're a much more professional organization.

Other middle management nurses support professional unionism and its singular focus on nursing rather than on multiple occupations that are seemingly unrelated in their concerns. Susan Stebbins, a middle manager from the oncology unit who has worked at St. John's for five and a half years, professes this view. Stebbins is a single woman who has lived a quiet life in Brooklyn. Her father was a career soldier who died when she was very young, and her mother taught in a parochial school. No one in her family was ever affiliated with any type of union, but she is impressed with NYSNA's focus on "polite behavior," which she feels is appropriate for white collar nurses. She supports the professional union's sole focus on nursing and credentialism and rejects trade unions for their class focus and their use of unnecessary muscle:

NYSNA is a professional organization. I think if nurses are gonna be unionized at all, it should be with a professional union. Many times [with a trade union], we had grievances where delegates from the union might be a radiology technician, being witness to a nurse [representing a nurse to management]. I don't feel technicians are on the same level as nurses and shouldn't be representing them.

1199 uses bullying tactics . . . a lot of yelling. The delegates would argue with the person doing the disciplinary action. They wouldn't try to work things out.

NYSNA, from the posture of the people there, was more concerned with what nursing is and what nurses hope to achieve. . . . Like with educational requirements, NYSNA was more willing to work things out, compromise with the administration. They'd say, "Well, we don't mind such and such; just keep us informed."

Other nurses in the medium class position were similarly single minded in their concern with "what nursing is" or "nursing practice" and the professional union's approach on this issue. "Nursing practice" can be translated into lay terms as the differentiation of manual from mental nursing work, and cementing this stratification into the occupation. Carin Whelehan, who has worked in the CCU at St. John's for two years, supports NYSNA's focus on the professional role of nursing. This approach seeks to eliminate nonnursing tasks, which "degrade" the occupation by saddling nurses with menial duties. She, like most other middle management nurses, climbed her way up the nursing educational ladder from a diploma to a master's in nursing. She describes her new role at the hospital as a middle manager with "expert power" and explains her support of NYSNA as follows:

NYSNA . . . has an understanding of the professional role of nurses. It concentrates on issues of professionalism like background educational preparation to practice [and] "non-nursing functions." The professional organization has more of an understanding of what is and what is not a nursing function.

This has always been an issue for us. If someone vomits, should the nurse or housekeeping clean it up? Or, picking up drugs—should the nurse or ancillary do it? Only a professional union deals with these issues.

Most middle management nurses, in their stalwart efforts to improve their status, appreciate the role that the professional union plays in cementing the widening fissures between nursing and other occupations. By promoting "dumping" of the more menial tasks onto the less skilled workers, NYSNA is seen as working toward elevating the status of nursing. These nurses choose to disassociate themselves from blue collar workers and often use a smokescreen for this separatist position by invoking the refrain, "Nurses have to be represented only by other nurses," because, the logic continues, "an organization made up of other occupations will never fully understand their needs."

Even Ronnie Blevins, the middle manager from Mt. Zion oncology unit who basked in the notion of mixing different classes, emphasized her desire to have nurses represented only by other nurses. She says:

Only nurses can understand the needs of other nurses. I believe we have to belong to our own professional organization. If it doesn't work, make it work. NYSNA is an organization of nurses, not teachers or longshoremen.

There are more issues to be solved than just a contract. The AFT or 1199 doesn't represent me as a nurse. It's not what I believe a professional person should be: having some class, some education and human dignity.

Likewise, Jean Omohundro, middle management nurse from Mt. Zion's medical-surgical unit, also expressed the desire for nurses to be represented only by other nurses. Oddly enough, both of these middle managers have been around Mt. Zion for over two decades and were willing to talk for hours about their lack of control over nursing work, their subordination to layers of administrators and physicians, and their sincere desire to implement change in the work conditions. Nevertheless, their implicit concern with personal freedom via credentialism and status won out. They do not want their occupation to be associated with less prestigious ones (at least from their vantage point). Jean Omohundro expressed it this way:

As nurses, our jobs and responsibilities are different. Let's say the Teamsters represent you. Most nurses don't even know what the hell a longshoreman is. Why should we go out on strike with them? We sure don't want longshoremen going out in sympathy for us, and we don't want to go out with them.

Other middle management nurses rejected common class interests with members of other occupations in favor of maintaining nursing as separate, thereby elevating its status as well. If raising the prestige of nursing meant firing nurses or enforcing credentialism, they supported it. Seena Rocco was very concerned about not "screwing her profession" by airing the dirty laundry with me, and she spoke from her managerial vantage point, emphasizing the professional union's ability to understand "nurses' needs," such as the necessity for staff nurses to perform extra work or take extra exams in order to practice in certain clinical areas. She was confident that NYSNA would support "nurses' need" (nursing management's need, that is) to fire any nurse deemed incompetent:

NYSNA is a professional organization. Nurses need to represent nurses. They conduct themselves in a professional manner where nurses would be proud to be represented by them.

NYSNA is concerned with the needs of professionals. They understand nursing in different areas of the hospital—that different specialties have certain tests that nurses have to pass to be able to work there. NYSNA wouldn't complain if nurses have to do extra

work or go through extra tests to work in a particular area. . . . They also understand if a nurse has to be terminated.

Seena Rocco clearly revealed that the professional union represents nursing management's priorities, not those of frontline nurses. According to her view, NYSNA does, and it should advocate for "nursing," not nurses, by "upholding the standards of nursing," over and above the interests of individual nurses. Once again, the middle manager blames the victim.

These middle managerial nurses champion professional unionism because it upholds the dominant segment of their conflicted interests, their managerial interests, reflected in the individualist aspect of their vision of professionalism: human capital. This vision, based on the culture of meritocracy, promotes cooperation with management, along with an enlarged fault line between frontline nurses and lower status occupations. Professional unionism does not, however, advance that other segment of their interests, their collective need, as subordinate employees, for control over the conditions of their work.

Only 6 percent, or 1 nurse out of 17 in the medium class position, supported trade unionism. The other 94 percent rejected it, primarily because, in their estimation, blue collar members of trade unions denigrate the white collar image of nursing they are trying to impart. Jackie Sauter, a middle manager at St. John's Hospital on the CCU, rejects trade unions for this reason. She feels they diminish the professional image of nurses by associating them with undesirable workers, weakening their toehold grip on prestige:

I think trade unions degrade the professional image of nursing. It lumps nurses together with nursing assistants and technicians. Since we're struggling to get and keep a professional image to the public, to doctors and everybody, there's no way we should belong to a trade union.

Other middle managers were just as explicit in their goal of disassociating themselves from the working class. Marley Connett, a middle manager from St. John's Hospital, notes that the problem at her own institution is that no one views her as a manager, because "to the rest of the world, a nurse is just a nurse," and that nurse is working class. Because of this association of nursing with the working class, managers like herself find it difficult to rise above the riffraff. She suggests that many nurses are in fact working class and simply follow in the trade union footsteps of their fathers and brothers, a cycle she is determined to break. Identifying with higher-status occupations should help do the trick, according to Connett:

Women, years ago, believed that to get ahead, they had to do what their fathers, uncles, and brothers did. They were union people and expected it of their daughters as nurses. It makes nurses feel that they're on parity with other people in trade unions: transporters, messengers, or housekeepers.

I don't feel those people are equal to nurses, but I'm always dealing with people who do [other nurses]. They don't feel their job is any more valuable or on a higher level than these other people. No one treats them as if it is; administration certainly doesn't. Nurses are still paid an hourly wage, not salaried, and many things that govern people represented by unions still govern nurses. But I still don't believe nurses belong there. They have to see themselves as better.

Despite their persistent pursuit of prestige, middle managerial nurses remain frustrated with their position as subordinate employees and their subsequent ineffectiveness in changing their conditions at work. They lack job security and are dissatisfied with their low salaries, minimal opportunity for advancement, and lack of grievance mechanisms.[5]

Conflicted Class Identity

Nurses in a medium class position are thus conflicted in their class identity. Jean Omohundro provides a clear example of such conflict. Although she lives a comfortable life outside work, she does not define herself as an "upper-class person." Her identity is based on her position at work. In fact she fought tooth and nail as a former head nurse to stay in the NYSNA bargaining unit because she felt nurses needed protection. In the early 1970s, she, along with other head nurses who were being upgraded out of the bargaining unit, "even went to Henry Van Arsdale of the United Federation of Teachers [UFT] for help," since "NYSNA was totally unresponsive."[6] UFT said there was nothing it could do. The primary issue for the head nurses at the time was job security. Omohundro felt then, and still feels now, that her job security is practically nil:

I wouldn't trust those ladies [nursing administrators] to save my neck one iota; . . . they'll can you in a minute. Anyway, they're all worried about their own necks right now--even though they'd never admit it. My number 1 reason for wanting the union [UFT or NYSNA] was job security.

When they changed our titles in 1976, from head nurse to clinical supervisor, their number 1 reason was to get us out of the union. We were in court for three months fighting them on this issue . . . to prove we didn't meet the category for supervisor. Obviously, we lost.

Ronnie Blevins similarly describes her insecurity on bread-and-butter issues such as job security, grievance mechanisms, and salary. These nurses are caught by their own conflicted class identity, however. Their contradictory position in the class structure and their conflicted cultural interpretation of that position leads them down a blind alley. Their individualist goals and individualist solutions, as

Gans (1988) warned, create victims by preventing them from seeking a viable collective solution to their collective problem. Blevins said:

My salary is very important to me. My time is valuable, and I should get what I'm worth. After 34 years of nursing I earn $40,000. My little niece, right out of business school, with an M.B.A., earns $40,000. Grievance procedures are important to me because they fire us according to how they want to. I have no recourse.

When social phenomena are described and explained in individualist terms (individual inadequacy, or crude "blue collar" behaviors), ties are loosened between those who are similarly situated, and as mid-level nurse Dawn Ford puts it, "It's nice to move up, but it becomes lonely and insecure." Ford is one of the few black women in any management tier at Mt. Zion. She exemplifies the problem nurses in a medium class position face. While not sure where the ax will fall in the light of the imminent layoffs, they are struggling to figure out some means to protect themselves. Pushed out of collective protection offered by the professional union, meager as it may have been, they are scrambling for some useful alternative. Dawn Ford is aware, however, that they are ultimately helpless without a union:

We're meeting today to decide what to do. . . . Not having a union, there's not much you can do. But in numbers we might be more effective. There are not too many jobs today, and they're closing units.
   They can call me tomorrow and say, "We're closing your unit in four weeks. I'm sorry but you'll have to leave," and that'll be that.

Successful collective action requires mutual trust, recognition of common interests, and some form of leverage, such as work stoppage, before disaster strikes. Without any of these characteristics, middle managers remain trapped by their own conflicted ideology. Insistent that they must remain separate from other low-ranking workers, they are isolated in their own time of need. No one expressed sympathy (strikes or otherwise) with these middle managerial nurses.
   Nevertheless, professional unionism, along with the ideology undergirding this strategy, is Sisyphean: no matter how hard nurses push for credentialism and prestige, their inability to determine the terms and conditions of their work continues to roll back on them due to their ultimately subordinate status as employees and their almost fanatical belief in individualism.

HIGH CLASS POSITION

In contrast to the middle managerial nurses' composite definition of professionalism (work control and popular individualism via the human capital strategy of credentialism), 80 percent of administrative nurses--those in high class locations--interpret professionalism as synonymous with capitalist individualism (pursuit of market control, maximum profits, and credentialism), drawing heavily, on the culture of meritocracy. While control over such conditions of work as job security, grievance procedures, stress, speed-up, unsafe conditions, and autonomy are important elements in the middle manager's concept of professionalism, they are not part of the administrative nurse's conceptual vision. Most of these work issues, aside from job security and authority, are in fact no longer part of their experience as administrative nurses. Twenty percent do, however, define professionalism as middle managerial nurses do: both work control and popular individualism, indicating a more contradictory class position for a minority of nurses in a high class position as well.

Larry Porta, an administrative nurse in the psychiatric unit at Mt. Zion, personifies the culture of meritocracy in his personal climb to success. He is African-American, originally from a poor, rural southern town, who started his career in health care as a hospital orderly. His father, a man of the cloth, had high aspirations for his children. Porta describes himself as attempting to fulfill his father's dreams. He was a superior student--valedictorian of his high school class, Phi Beta Kappa in college--yet initially unable to get into nursing school and never able to break the barriers for entrance into medical school during the 1950s. After my persistent probing, he finally gave credence to the possibility that the roadblocks he encountered with entrance into professional school may have been due to racial discrimination. (Despite his high grade point average he was never admitted into medical school, and all but one nursing school had rejected him.) Nevertheless, like Supreme Court justice Clarence Thomas, Porta claims to have picked himself up by the bootstraps and pursued credentialism and compliance with the powers that be as his tickets to success:

My father was a minister, and he preset the goals for me and my nine brothers and sisters. He wanted us to be upwardly mobile. . . .
   I used to be a hospital orderly. They liked me there; they could tell I had ambitions. Now I'm a nursing administrator. Two years out of school, they promoted me from staff nurse to supervisor. . . .
   [Professionalism is] showing good judgment, not talking back, taking responsibility for what you're supposed to do, and getting a baccalaureate degree.

Porta equates professionalism with upward mobility and upward mobility with meritocracy. In his mind, cultivating his human capital and fitting in with the power structure is the only way to rise in the occupational structure. Ameliorating the conditions of work, significant in the interpretation of professionalism for nurses in both the low and medium class positions, does not enter his horizon. Rising to the top as an individual, relying on his own cleverness and human capital improvements to reap the greatest personal windfall, is paramount to Porta.

The emphasis on educational credentialism and "proper behavior" as antecedents of upward mobility clearly transcend nursing and extend into much of

20th-century life. This interpretation of professionalism, far more than the previous two, encompasses the general principles of individualism, lock, stock, and barrel, placing each individual as solely responsible for his or her own station in life. While many of society's ills have been attributed to this philosophy (the overwhelming selfishness, materialism, and "loss of community" in American culture) (Bellah, 1985), nurses in a high class location are most absorbed by it. They generally deem these characteristics as part of the natural, Social Darwinist order of things. Porta subscribes to these principles and struggled to achieve not only credentialism but also integration into the dominant (white) professional culture he found there. He feels his climb up the ladder of success rested not only on his qualifications but on his personal qualities, particularly his chameleon-like ability to exude predominantly white, middle-class values. He worked to overcome his racial and class background and taught himself to mix with the white culture:

I am middle class, which I determine by my social position. Socially I am black. I grew up down South, and we were not well off by any means. I taught myself to mingle multiracially and socioculturally. I am black, but I am able to appreciate the racial and cultural components of white culture, Hispanic culture, black culture. . . . I appreciate arts and science, ballet and opera, soul music. . . . I can communicate with different people, but I do best with the middle class. . . . I consider myself middle class.[7]

Porta professes the individualist doctrine held by the majority of nurses in a high class position. Better thy self, not the hierarchical, degraded health care structure in which nurses in a high-class position are embedded--that is, professionalism. Those with ability who keep their nose to the grindstone, according to this view, can succeed and attain the American dream. Competition will naturally weed out the incompetent. Structural phenomena, such as institutional racism, which may have prohibited Porta from attending the schools of his choice, and ultimately his career choice, do not fit into the picture.

The vice president of nursing at St. John's Hospital, whose job has more to do with running a business than it does with nursing per se, defines professionalism according to similar tenets. Charlotte Ramsey purports that nurses will strengthen their autonomy and chances for occupational advancement by improving their personal traits and credentials, a path she has followed. She started out 30 years ago with a diploma in nursing (which she attained through a hospital apprenticeship program) followed by a master's in public administration. Although she has worked in her vice presidential capacity for only three years, her vision of professionalism affirms the principles of blame-the-victim individualism:

Professionalism is autonomy, accountability and responsibility. . . . We hope that by taking responsibility, improving their expertise, our nurses will become more autonomous, more professional.

She then intimated that nurses with educational credentials will also exhibit compliant behavior, more in line with her needs as a vice president:

We're starting to get more powerful. I don't want dumb, uneducated nurses. The dumb ones, not the smart ones, shoot their mouths off.

For Charlotte Ramsey, improper behavior, which stems from a lack of education (and the "wrong" class background), is antithetical to professionalism. Better-educated nurses are superior workers, the only ones capable of performing a heavier workload, while maintaining a less hostile posture to management's increasing demands. Although non-college-educated nurses have constituted the majority of the nursing labor force until this decade, the vice president feels hospitals will be unable to function without college-educated nurses in the future. She argues that the newer form of hospital reimbursement, DRGs, will demand the skills of college-educated nurses. This form of reimbursement, in which third-party insurers, both public and private, reimburse hospitals a set fee for given diseases and procedures (rather than leaving it up to the discretion of the physician as occurred in the past), reduces the amount of time patients stay in the hospital. Ramsey argues that only college-educated nurses will be able to function with the necessary speed and skill in this new process (more susceptible to managerial control, without work stoppages):

With DRGs, only RNs with baccalaureates will be able to get the patient out the fastest. They'll be able to do the proper assessment of the patient and give the best care. . . . Only a B.S.N. can assess the patient in a timely fashion. They can integrate all the ser-vices . . . home care, social services. . . . Only RNs are educated enough to assume those functions.
Some think auxiliaries are a cheaper and more efficient way of doing it, so hire all auxiliary workers. We think not.

Ramsey maintains that college-educated nursing staff are better providers of care (less resistant to authority), and she has the power to make her beliefs stick.[8] In 1980 she laid off most of the lower-status auxiliary nursing workers in her hospital (nursing aides and LPNs), many of whom had been employed there for over 20 years.

Patty Cilantro, the director of continuing education and one of the vice president's senior administrators at St. John's, explained somewhat defensively that these less prestigious nursing workers were not fired but laid off because they were no longer the most "qualified resource" available:

We never *terminated* LPNS or aides. It was a layoff. We were interested in an all-RN staff. . . . Get the biggest bang for your buck. . . . You want the highest qualified resource.

Thus, in the name of a higher-quality (and a more compliant) workforce, these administrative nurses, demanding higher educational credentials and "proper behavior" from their staff, are attempting to uplift the status of their occupation by eliminating the undereducated, lower-status nurses who complain about the conditions of their work. Such a strategy is merely a continuation of the process that nursing administrators and educators had begun in the late 1800s. They were attempting to rid the occupation of its working-class members through the "objective" weeding-out process of increased credentialism.

Since the capitalist individualist ideology of professionalism draws on the culture of meritocracy and assumes that those who have the ability to improve their human capital will, and those who do not will not, the administrative nurses feel justified in discarding nurses who remain on the lower rungs of the status ladder (as they have less ambition and, according to this perspective, less ability).

While the occupation can gain status by ridding itself of its less educated (and working-class) members, individual nurses must contribute to elevating its prestige through credentialism. Melon McGill, who has worked in an administrative nursing capacity at Mt. Zion for two and a half years, expressed this view. She has been a nurse for 19 years but within the first five minutes of our conversation wanted to discuss only her credentialism: the number of degrees, partial degrees, and areas of expertise she had gained from her recent schooling. Ironically, she explained that nurses used to feel insecure about their status since they lacked true "expertise." Now, however, nursing has its own theories and presumably has overcome its insecurity about a body of knowledge it can claim as its own:

Nursing used to have a problem with its identity. Physical therapists do this, physicians do that, but what do we do? We used to feel insecure. We really were the handmaidens to physicians. Now we have our own theories.

McGill believes nursing need not be so threatened by its diminutive status in contrast to medicine now that it has its own professional associations, journals, and conventions. She illustrates this point even further by rattling off a litany of costly organizations to which she belongs:

As a professional I belong to different professional organizations. . . . I've just been appointed to the board of directors of the American Association of Neuro Science Nurses. . . . We sponsor a major convention every year which focuses on the education of nurses. . . .

I'm also a member of other professional organizations. . . . It costs me a fortune to belong. . . . The American Heart Association, Sigma Theta Ta, the National Honor Society for Nurses, and the ANA. The ANA alone costs me $200 a year. I spend between $300 and $400 a year. . . . With most of these organizations, it seems like all we do is spend years meeting.

Thus, like all other fledgling disciplines, nursing is seeking a circumscribed body of knowledge to call its own, developing journals and holding expensive conferences. In addition to enhancing status, the executives' interpretation of professionalism incorporates a service ethic that enjoins nurses to replace their own needs with those of their patients (Larson, 1977; Edwards, 1979). This philosophy cum policy, a twist on nurses' altruistic devotion to helping others, generally compels nurses to comply with management's need for cheap labor. After explaining that nurses are frequently obliged to work double shifts (overtime) and request payment for that overtime, McGill expresses dismay at their request. Professionals should not put a price tag on the number of hours they work. Rather, their commitment to patients should supersede their own "selfish need" for money:

Nurses want to be treated as professionals but work by rules that aren't professional. . . . [For example], it's the end of the shift and they're not finished with patient care yet. They say, "Will I get paid for it?"

We say that's conflictual. We try to say to them you do it because you're a professional. They say they want to get paid. To me, that is blue collar. . . . Anyway, to pay a nurse time and a half to work a double shift is just not in our best interest.

Ironically, McGill, like the mid-level nurses, is ensnared by her own view of professionalism. She expressed chagrin about getting paid for her own overtime because it is unprofessional. Nevertheless, she admitted she would be feebleminded to give up her overtime pay. Thus, the capitalist individualist ideology of professionalism, internalized by the administrative nurses themselves, acts as a form of control over them as well:

I've never put a price tag on the number of hours I work. I've never asked for overtime, and I've never asked for comp [pay for working overtime] time. I'm sort of embarrassed by it. It's not professional.

When the staff was on strike, I worked here until 11 every night. I didn't ask for comp time. But, I tell you, I took it. I'd be a fool not to. It's too bad the system is that way, though, because its really not professional.

Not only does this vision of professionalism trap McGill into feeling embarrassed, but it also affects her attitude toward her own job security. Like Fortune 500 executives who blame themselves for their "fall from grace," as they become subject to corporate downsizing (layoffs) (Newman, 1988), McGill adopts the perspective of self-sacrifice and takes personal responsibility for the structural problems she confronts at work. She looks within herself for individual solutions to her own probable layoff, a collective problem facing all managers in the hospital. Individuals are held responsible for their own destinies according to this perspective; hence, individuals must make amends for their own failures:

I have no union to support me, and there's a strong possibility that they might just cut my position. I think it's all a part of growing up. Life just isn't always fair. I don't think they'd really listen to me if I had a problem anyway. So I'll probably go back to school-- become a lawyer or get involved with the health corporations. If they're hiring people to make megabucks, it might as well be me.

Penny McCarthy, an administrative nurse who has worked at St. John's for the past three years as director of recruitment and retention, is in the same boat as McGill. She is busy promoting nurses' "altruistic responsibility" to patients and admonishing her subordinates not to engage in strikes because they are unprofessional, selfish actions, removing nurses from their primary commitment to public service (the hospital). Nevertheless, she too is worried about the security of her own job:

Professionalism means educating yourself and conducting yourself responsibly. Self-interest can be good, but we all have to remember what we entered the profession for: commitment to our patients. So when you take an action like a strike, you are neglecting your commitment; it's being selfish and unprofessional.
I might lose my own job. But what shall I do? Strike? Not on your life.

As members of administration, nurses in a high class position identify with the administrative, Social Darwinist analysis of life: expend energy on improving one's self, not the institution, for it's survival of the fittest out there. They incorporate human capital into their collective conscience, perceived as the token for entry into the high-status white collar world. Hence, compliant behaviors, credentialism, and the culture of meritocracy supersede views of their own, as well as of their subordinates', less-than-ideal work conditions. Although staff-patient ratios, shift work, and overtime pay are not as crucial to these nurses as their own job security and limits on their authority, their primary focus within the workplace is internal: changing themselves, not the hospital. Indeed, bread-and-butter issues are defined by administrative nurses as unprofessional, while total commitment to professional service (the employer) is the high-status, white collar preoccupation.

Choosing Collective Strategy: The Best Way Up

The collective strategy that aims to realize the capitalist individualist interpretation of professionalism focuses on collective efforts for change outside the workplace, in the government arena. Unlike professional unionism, which promotes broader cultural values of individualism (improving one's human capital) with control over work conditions, professionalization ignores immediate issues of control over conditions of work.   In contrast, professionalization addresses control over nursing issues at the political level of the state.

Professionalization is a general strategy in which the elites of nursing attempt to gain monopoly control over both the education and practice of the occupation. The nursing educators and administrators--those nurses in a high class position-- constitute the elite, which seeks monopoly control over nursing education and practice through the licensure process. Indeed, they have lobbied hard for the Entry into Practice Proposal, an amendment to the education law in New York State that would require all nurses to attain a baccalaureate degree from a four-year college and all associate nurses to attain an associate degree from a two-year community college (Article 139 of the Higher Education Law State of New York, 1983).

While the overt rationale for this act is to "clarify and standardize" the education and practice of nursing so as to "eliminate public confusion" (NYSNA, 1983), this is clearly a smokescreen for their desire to rid the occupation of its undereducated, working class members. As Andrew Dolan states, "There has never been any evidence that public confusion exists. It is unlikely that the public even knows that there are three educational pathways to RN licensure. . . . If the public is confused about anything, it is probably about the difference between RNs and LPNs, a distinction which the 1985 Proposal [retitled the Entry into Practice Act], perpetuates (Dolan, 1979b: 511).

Nevertheless, the vice president of nursing at St. John's, Charlotte Ramsey, employs this very rationale in her support of professionalization:

It's been multiple confusion for everyone with nurses educated at diploma, associate degree, and B.S.N. level. They all function as professionals, yet they aren't all equal. Having technical and professional nurses separated out [proposed by the entry into practice bill] will clarify the situation for everyone.

The real intent of this legislation is to professionalize nursing: gain control over the supply, demand, and economic rewards for nurses. Nurses in a high class location seek to become the gatekeepers for the occupation, controlling the professional schools, which guard entrance to the occupation. Once monopoly control is accomplished, nursing can achieve (it is hoped) the prize in health care occupations: independence rendered by fee for service. Joann Pfeil, an administrative nurse at St. John's for the past two and a half years, equates professionalism with this entrepreneurial medical model, a capitalist individualist construction:

Professionalism means getting fee for service. It would give us the power, salaries, and credibility [with] the public we deserve.
    The physicians have the AMA, and it has power. We need to organize to be professionals with power like that. As its stands, nurses don't have power or credibility with the public.

In addition to gaining market control over the occupation in order to maximize power and profits, many argue this strategy is also an attempt to conceal and legitimate inequality within the occupation. By creating and mandating a requisite body of expertise for practice through an accredited institution of higher learning, such educational standards become an "objective" criteria sieve (e.g., entry exams or qualifications) through which certain classes and ethnic groups will likely not pass (Larson, 1977; Dolan, 1979b; Cohen, 1979; Collins, 1979).[9]

Embodied within this vision of professionalism is also a rather virulent anti-unionism, which is once again considered detrimental to the white collar image of nursing. Melon McGill states this position clearly:

I am not favorable toward bargaining status for nurses at all. . . . I really feel bargaining units identify us as blue collar. It creates role confusion. Nurses want to be professionals yet are forced by the union to work by rules that are unprofessional. For example, in one unit, they can't make independent decisions about patient care because they're afraid of how they'll be thought of by the bargaining unit.

This, of course, is the antithesis of the view held by most nurses in a low class position concerning their lack of autonomy. They attribute it to union weakness, not union strength. Nurses in a high class location, however, view trade unionism as a challenge to their administrative authority. This threat to their managerial control is transmuted into yet another variation of professionalism. Not only does trade unionism diminish the white collar image they are trying to preserve, but it also solidifies work rules such as limits on mandated overtime (double shifts), once again encroaching on their managerial privilege. Larry Porta expresses these views:

Trade unions are a blue collar orientation. They don't understand the way professionals work. Professionals don't need a contract. They don't need to put things in writing. Just a verbal agreement is enough.

A professional person should complete the job as it is intrinsically presented to them. They shouldn't think of themselves as 7 to 3:30 workers. . . . They should work until the job is done and not ask for overtime. Professionals are committed first to their practice as defined by the legislature and your educational influences. Trade unions don't understand this.

Other administrative nurses went even further in their explicit dislike of trade unions. Patty Cilantro, through a slip of the tongue, implicated her administration in its dismantling of the League of Registered Nurses, 1199.

I have strong negative feelings about trade unions. I don't think any trade union has ever identified the professional image of the nurse. 1199 doesn't even know what a professional nurse is and has no desire to know. . . . We decertified them. . . . I, I mean *they* decertified 1199. Its hard to decertify a union. NLRB wasn't happy; they investigated us in depth. 1199 is a fanatical union. One nurse was raped, another person was knifed during the strike. Can I prove that those were 1199 phone calls harassing the nurses? No, not necessarily.

Eighty percent of the administrative nurses view the ideology of professionalism as pure capitalist individualism, enhancing individual human capital and gaining market control over the occupation to achieve economic and social status.

By controlling nursing education and practice, these nurses believe the greatest profits will come to those whose strengths are most deserving. In addition, they incorporate the service ethic into their definition to promote compliance with management. Finally, they denigrate trade unionism as an inviolate measure of nonprofessionalism. The strategy of professionalization embodies capitalist individualist values yet necessitates collective actions to achieve them.

CONCLUSION

Nurses reveal their class interests through their ideology of professionalism. Each group fashions a version that fits its experience in the workplace and thus provides authoritative concepts. This transformed, redefined ideology, intimately related to adoption or rejection of the broader cultural constructs of meritocracy and individualism, then became the goal around which nurses in each class position collectively organized, "making [their] autonomous politics possible" (Geertz, 1973: 220).

Nurses in the low class position (84 percent), reshaped professionalism into an ideology that connotes work control: greater control over conditions of their work, rewarded by greater salary, dignity, and security on the job. They incorporate the Protestant work ethic into their cultural understanding of professionalism. Being unrewarded, and in fact castigated for what they perceive to be laudatory qualities (hard work, altruism, and skill), led them to view the workplace as a contested terrain where they, as employees, collectively contested management's encroachment on their rights. Through their interpretation of professionalism, they conveyed their class identity, as workers, in search of a "real" union to protect their workplace interests. The political tactic that emerged from their interpretation of professionalism was cooperative economic struggle in the workplace, culminating in the strategy of trade unionism. Although in reality they may not have elected a trade union, the majority of nurses expressed an ideology and collective strategy in concert with the collective ideals of trade unionism.

In contrast, 76 percent of nurses in the medium class position, occupying a more contradictory class position, have a more complex interpretation of professionalism, which included both work control and popular individualism. They incorporate the values of meritocracy as it permeates American work culture, in combination with work control, into their vision of professionalism. Their class identity is mixed, resulting from their dual role as employees and managers; yet the strongest pull is from management, given that it has institutionalized these middle managerial positions into the upper echelons of the hospital authority structure. Nurses in this class position perceive their inability to attain their individual goals as linked to their own personal shortcomings, as well as the conflict between nursing and other occupations. The strategy that 94 percent of these nurses support is professional unionism. Although they are no longer eligible for membership in the collective bargaining unit, they support the professional association's individualist strategy of credentialism, as well as minimal economic struggle within the workplace (compromising with hospital management as much as possible). Thus, professional unionism represents the individualist goals of middle managers and recognizes their lack thereof.

Finally, 80 percent of the nurses in the high class position interpret professionalism as synonymous with capitalist individualism. Social and economic status can be attained only by those individuals who choose a twofold approach: (1) improving their own human capital through credentialism and compliant behaviors, in concert with the goals of management, and (2) gaining monopoly control over the education and market of the occupation. They view the nature of conflict as that between different occupations, which is fought outside the workplace, in state and federal arenas. Thus, they focus on securing greater occupational turf, power, and profits by pressuring state and federal legislatures.

The collective strategy that reflects this interpretation of professionalism is professionalization: monopoly control over the occupation's expertise, producers of that expertise, and market for that expertise. All nurses in the high class location supported this strategy. Through such an "objective," gatekeeper's strategy, nurses in the high class position conceal and legitimate inequality in their occupation, social and economic superiority for the nursing elite, revealing their own class identification with the powers that be.

NOTES

1.   As I discussed in Chapter 1, nurses at each research site had actively worked to decertify their bargaining representatives. St. John's nurses successfully decertified the League of Registered Nurses, Local 1199 in 1984 in favor of NYSNA, and Mt. Zion nurses unsuccessfully attempted to decertify NYSNA in 1982 in favor of Local 1199 of the National Union of Hospital and Health Care Employees, League of Registered Nurses or the Federation of Nurses/AFT. NYSNA won 53 percent of the vote at Mt. Zion, with the trade unions winning 43 percent of the vote. Four percent of the votes were challenged. At St. John's Hospital, NYSNA won.

2.   This information was disseminated by management in a memo, which took a stab against the American Federation of Teachers (AFT) by associating it with the tough-guy image of trade unionism. The union appears to have been deliberately mislabeled, "The United Federation of Teachers, AFL/CIO." The correct title is Federation of Nurses/AFT.

3.   Attributing this rather high salary to the blue collar labor force makes sense when considering that she works on a daily basis with physicians and administrators who earn well over three times this amount.

4.   Incorporating the dissemination of human capital ideology into the job description of nurses in a medium class location is in concert with E. O. Wright's analysis of class alliances. He argues that dominant classes pursue class alliances with

contradictory class locations in order to neutralize their potential threat by tying their interests together (E. O. Wright, 1989: 30).

5.   The middle managers who had worked at either St. John's or Mt. Zion hospital in the former capacity of head nurse, before the position was eliminated and upgraded to clinical nurse specialist, nursing care coordinator, or clinical nursing supervisor, with real supervisory duties, fought the hospital's decision to remove them from the professional union's bargaining unit.

6.   The NYSNA executive committee, comprising elected Mt. Zion staff nurses, had filed an unfair labor practice charge against the hospital when it attempted to remove head nurses from the bargaining unit and revamp their positions into supervisory jobs. (The hospital removed them from the bargaining unit because these head nurse positions had been transformed into "statutory supervisors," effectively participating in hiring, firing, promotion, grievances, and creation of policy.) The executive committee charged the hospital with refusing to deal with the terms and conditions of employment of persons holding the disputed new title of clinical and administrative supervisor, since, as head nurses (their previous titles), they were still covered by their previous contract. Meanwhile, the NYSNA representative for Mt. Zion Hospital, was secretly undermining these actions. While appearing to fight the hospital-sending literature to the members that explained what the hospital was doing to the head nurses, she had already, on December 12, 1976, reached a secret agreement with the hospital that NYSNA would withdraw its unfair labor practice charge. NYSNA agreed, unbeknown to the Mt. Zion NYSNA executive committee, that these titles may be removed from the bargaining unit under the following conditions: "As long as the New York State Nurses Association is the exclusive bargaining representative for nurses at Mt. Zion, the hospital will not allege that any other titles are 'statutory supervisors,' nor will they initiate any actions to exclude other titles from the bargaining unit" (NYSNA Memo to Executive Vice President for Personnel from Deputy Director of NYSNA, December 8, 1976: 1). The Mt. Zion nurses involved were incensed by NYSNA's actions.

7.   Larry Porta, the administrative nurse from the psychiatry division at Mt. Zion, was so adept in promoting compliance with management that after 22 years at the hospital, he transferred this skill to another job, with a life insurance company. His new duties were focused on revamping the values and behaviors of minority employees. He would teach them to internalize the dominant values of the company. He said, "I'm going to be the director of the 'psycho social development committee' at Equitable Life Insurance. I'll work with their employees and teach them that the employee must be a chameleon and change to meet the values of the company. . . . I'll work especially with black employees and teach them to adopt the values and culture of the company and their clients."

8.   This view is contrary to the generally accepted perception that college-educated nurses lack hospital experience and are thus less adept in providing care for the patients, compared to associate degree and diploma nurses whose education consists of at least some hospital apprenticeship.

9.   Sarfatti Larson makes this point in more general terms: "Professionalization [is] the process by which producers of special services sought to constitute and control a market for their 'expertise.' . . . Professionalization appears also as a collective assertion of special social status and . . . upward social mobility. In other words, the constitution of professional markets which began in the 19th-century inaugurated a new form of structured inequality. . . . The restructuring of social inequality in contemporary

capitalist societies is the occupational hierarchy . . . a differential system of competencies and rewards; [its] legitimacy is founded on the achievement of socially recognized expertise or, more simply, on a system of education and credentialing. . . .

"Professionalism has [also] become an ideology, not only an image which consciously inspires collective or individual efforts, but a mystification which unconsciously obscures real social structures and relations" (Larson, 1977: xvi-xviii).

Chapter 5

Conclusion (or Where Does the Frayed Collar Go From Here?)

This study sought to determine the way in which educated, salaried, white collar workers respond to their conditions of work in large bureaucratic organizations and attempts to analyze the political and cultural coherence of that response. As representatives of the growing ranks of white collar service workers, nurses might display a unified force for substantial social change (class consciousness), as was expected at one time from American industrial workers.

Such an investigation emerged within the debate on how to characterize these workers objectively. They are often casually referred to as professionals since segments of white collar workers are so classified by the U.S. Bureau of Labor Statistics. An analytic problem arises, however, as many social scientists argue such workers do not fit the accepted definition of professional: workers generally distinguished by their privilege and autonomy, derived from lengthy training and expertise (Hughes, 1958).

Many theorists have argued that contemporary professional workers no longer have the privilege and autonomy of their predecessors. That is, professionals in the past were characterized as independent entrepreneurs, able to deliver their services directly to their clients, with no intermediary. Today, however, most educated, white collar workers are salaried, and they are employed by large, bureaucratic organizations, which subjects, them to the authority and management of others. Many social scientists therefore argue that such workers are "proletarianized" as bureaucratic structures engender an increased division of labor, fragmenting their work into narrow specialization, and subordination to a centralized hierarchical authority. Edwards (1979), for example, argued that white collar workers are subject to an invisible form of bureaucratic control, in which management governs their work, supervision, and promotion through detailed written rules and policies, thus depriving them of autonomy. O'Connor (1973) and Oppenheimer (1975) hold that such workers who are employed in the public sector (e.g., education, medicine, and social services) are particularly vulnerable to proletarianization since their labor is subject to cutbacks as public coffers contract or public priorities change. Such public sector workers, always threatened by budget crises, are increasingly subject to managerial forms of control traditionally applied to private sector industrial workers.

Others have characterized educated, wage-earning white collar workers as members of a "new working class" (Gorz, 1967; Touraine, 1971; Mallet, 1975). They argue that although such workers may have control over their immediate technology, they still lack control over the management, use, and creative direction of their work.

Still others have generated yet another category for this group, the professional-managerial class (PMC) (Ehrenreich and Ehrenreich, 1979). These theorists place educated, dependent, white collar workers between management and labor, arguing that they share conditions of work with labor while performing social control functions of management.

Finally, other theorists claim these workers have increased privilege and autonomy. Most notably Friedson (1970, 1973a) has suggested that these educated white collar workers exercise great power in the large bureaucratic organizations that employ them. The power professionals wield is distinct from administrators of bureaucratic organizations, given their expertise. Bell (1973) has also argued that these educated, salaried white collar workers exercise great control in their organizations as most of production in the postindustrial society depends on scientific and technical knowledge, imbuing such workers with power. I suggest these characterizations provide inaccurate assessments of the objective class position of these workers. They do not all have the same quality or quantity of expertise and therefore do not all have comparable levels of power within, or for that matter outside, the organization.

Beyond a structural analysis on class position, theorists have also focused on the subjective dimension of these workers' lives. They have attempted to explain the discontent and potential for collective action among white collar workers. Various indexes for discontent have been utilized, but the two major ones are surveys on job satisfaction and incidence of unionization. One national survey, Quality of Employment Survey (Survey Research Center, 1977), demonstrated discontent among professionals, finding that such workers are more dissatisfied in their work than nonprofessionals regarding bread-and-butter issues (fringe benefits, job security, hours of work, health and safety, and the physical conditions in which they are employed) (SRC, 1977). Fantasia (1988) has argued that such attitudinal surveys as the Quality of Employment Survey (1977) are unable to capture the inherently contradictory, conflicted nature of the subjective dimension.

Other theorists have asserted that increased unionization among white collar workers indicates their potential for social change. Oppenheimer (1975), for example, argued that professional associations are being forced by their members to function more like labor unions and engage in collective bargaining. Others believe that trade unionism will increase, especially among public sector professionals, as fiscal crises at the level of the state increase (O'Connor, 1973). Gorz (1967) and Mallet (1975) think that professionals will organize into labor unions in order to gain more control over their work.[1]

Others have been less optimistic about professionals' potential for collective action. Mills (1951), for example, felt that white collar workers were too concerned with differentiating their status from blue collar workers and would therefore exhibit less of a tendency toward unionism. Bell (1973) portrayed these workers as having no need for labor unions given their monopoly over scientifically based skills and knowledge, enhancing their overall power. Derber (1982) argues that professionals subscribe to individualist values, prohibiting them from engaging in collective organizing at work.

This study has contributed to this debate by providing an empirical analysis of both the objective position and the subjective interests of one group of that educated, wage-earning white collar sector: nurses. By examining the nursing labor processes at Mt. Zion and St. John's hospitals, different segments within the occupation emerge, each with a distinct level of control in the workplace. More specifically, by employing Wright's concept of contradictory class locations (Wright, 1976) and analyzing nurses' levels of economic, political, and ideological control within the labor process, it became evident that nurses, though commonly defined as a single profession, occupy distinctly different class positions. Some have more control over their work than others.

One group of low-status nurses resembles blue collar industrial workers, another segment bears a resemblance to managerial work, and the middle-level nursing managers resemble both industrial workers and management. Nurses therefore represent an example of an educated, wage-earning, white collar profession, that is stratified into different class positions.

The three different class positions that became apparent within nursing are delineated here as simply high, medium, and low (in an effort to remain unentangled in the imbroglio of the exact constitution of the proletariat, petite bourgeoisie, and bourgeoisie). High class position refers to workers with high levels of control over the economic (division of labor), the ideological (conception and execution), and the political (supervisory hierarchy) domains in their work. Medium class position refers to workers with both high and low levels of control in these areas of their work. Finally, low class position refers to workers with low levels of control in the economic, political, and ideological aspects of their work.

Correlated with these three different class positions are three different interpretations of the professional, a ubiquitous ideology in the culture of nursing, and indeed, in America's overall work culture as well. By analyzing nurses' different interpretations of this ideology, I was able to view expressions of their class identity. The traditional 19th-century professional possessed the wholesome attributes of expertise, autonomy, and altruism. This professional was also an independent entrepreneur, upholding notions of meritocracy and individualism. Nurses in each class position reinterpret this embodiment of professionalism differently, in a manner that gives meaning to their own workplace experiences. Interpretations of this ideology therefore speak to the substantial differences in the conditions of work they face, the goals toward which they aspire, and the class alliances they seek. Nurses' class identity and class actions are thus revealed through an investigation of this ideology.

The majority of nurses in a low class position (84 percent) reinterpret the ideology of professionalism to mean greater work control (control over the conditions of their work as a reward for their altruism and devotion to the service ethic). In addition, 60 percent of these nurses support the collectivist strategy of trade unionism as the means to attain their vision of professionalism. Seventy-six percent of the nurses in a medium class position reinterpret the ideology of professionalism to mean both work control and popular individualism (individual freedom from economic, ideological, and political constraints in the workplace, through credentialism and compliance with management). Ninety-four percent of the nurses in this class position support the strategy of professional unionism as the means to attain their more mixed goals of increased control at work and greater social and economic status. Eighty percent of the nurses in a high class position interpret the ideology of professionalism to mean capitalist individualism (profit maximization through credentialism and market control over the occupation), and 60 percent support the strategy of professionalization to attain their vision.

By examining the ideology of professionalism I was able to gain a greater understanding of the different and sometimes overlapping worldviews that emerged with each class location. Indeed, it enabled me to "translate [their] sentiment into significance," as suggested by Geertz (1973), and examine that point of intersection in which shared perceptions become translated into political action.

The examination of the link between ideology in formation and class practice is part and parcel of a body of literature in the anthropology and sociology of work, along with social history, that has focused on work culture: the relationship between ideology and practice in the workplace. Triggered by Braverman's colossal study in 1974, which analyzed the degradation of industrial and service work in the 19th and early 20th centuries, scholars have since been trying to gain a better grasp of the active role that workers themselves have played in this process. Burawoy (1978) provided a noted critique of Braverman's failure in this area. In his study of shop floor life at Allied Corporation, Burawoy showed how the labor process itself "manufactured consent" among its workers (Burawoy, 1979). Some authors have studied the relationship between a worker's indigenous culture and the way it manifests itself in his or her actions in the workplace (Hareven and Vinovski, 1975; Gutman, 1976; Hareven, 1982; Sacks, 1984; Lamphere, 1985). Others have focused on the varied forms of worker resistance and informal relationships, shared values, and symbolic systems that emerge on shop floors, in department stores, hospitals, offices, and even in unemployment (Melosh, 1982; Benson, 1984; Shapiro-Perl, 1984; Sacks, 1988; Newman, 1986,

1988).

This literature perceives work cultures as live, fluid, reactive, and proactive expressions. It does not accept workers as simple sponges, absorbing the dominant cultural values of American individualism and narcissism. Rather, work cultures imbibe and transform aspects of the dominant culture, reaching into broader biblical, republican, and individualist roots--as Bellah (1985) argues-- and, as I suggest, infusing it with class-based meaning. Fantasia refers to these expressions as "cultures of solidarity . . . arising in conflict, creating and sustaining solidarity in opposition to the dominant structure" (Fantasia, 1988: 19).

This study has found that the work culture among nurses, conveyed through their interpretations of the dominant cultural symbol of the professional, is intimately tied to its antecedents in the broader cultural framework of American individualism. Bellah describes the origins of individualism as linked to early American traditions. While contemporary Americans applaud a just and compassionate society, the meaning of these concepts is varied. For some, a caring, fair society is bound up in the biblical, republican tradition, where "moral freedom" reigns: individuals do only that which is good, for the benefit of the larger community. Others interpret such a society in the utilitarian individualist tradition, where individuals are free to compete on the open market for their own materialist goals. Finally, according to Bellah, others interpret such a society in the expressive individualist tradition, where individuals are free to pursue sensual, intellectual, and emotional expression (Bellah et al., 1985).

When professionalism is viewed in its historic, cultural context, the significance and varied visions of it become more apparent. For some, a true professional is morally obligated to contribute expertise to the greater good and collectively struggle to realize that goal. For others, true professionalism means personal freedom through individualist means, for individualist goals. And for others, professionalism signifies more than personal freedom, but maximal profits, power, and prestige for the "most worthy."

In order to understand varied work cultures, we must go beyond connecting cultural meaning to its historic tradition. I suggest that the link must also be drawn between work culture and an analysis of the labor processes in which these workers are embedded, which, I have argued, contributes to the formation of their divergent ideologies and collective strategies. Most studies on work culture have alluded to but not empirically demonstrated this highly significant relationship.

This study has shown that a closer look at the historically specific relationship between labor process and the formation of ideology provides a sharper picture of the politics of a particular class location. This cannot always be discerned by merely examining the collective strategy actually chosen by a particular class position, however. As Edwards put it, the workplace is a "contested terrain" (Edwards, 1979), and management fights back with an array of managerial techniques that range from sophisticated anti-union strategies to the use of professionalism as a coercive anti-union tool. Trade unions themselves may be in a state of disarray as well, as was the case with the National Union of Health and Hospital Workers, Local 1199, in 1984. The complexity of this issue became apparent when 60 percent of the nurses in a low class position supported trade unionism and 84 percent of them defined the ideology of professionalism in terms of work control, yet neither hospital was represented by a union.

The criticism leveled against the studies in social history and the sociology and anthropology of work also applies to the new class professional and proletarianization theorists discussed earlier, who were partially correct in their subjective analyses of the white collar worker. Their inaccuracy lies in their class analyses. They mistook one segment of the white collar workforce for its totality. That is, they analyzed one piece of the white collar workforce as though it represented all white collar workers. Their analyses of the subjective dimension similarly focus on only one segment of this educated, white collar workforce as well. The analysis put forth by Gorz (1967) and Mallet (1975), for example, that professional workers will organize along the lines of labor unionism for greater control over the conditions of their work, applies to white collar workers in low class positions. Mills's (1951) analysis that professional workers lack but desire greater autonomy at work, while remaining overly concerned with differentiating themselves from blue collar workers, describes the views of white collar workers in medium class positions, who occupy the most contradictory class location. These workers I showed, support the strategy of professional unionism that alleges to provide both control over the conditions of work and increased status. Finally, the analysis put forth by Bell (1973), that educated, white collar workers have no need for labor unions due to their increased power derived from their scientifically based skills and knowledge, as well as that of Derber (1982), that white collar workers have imbibed individualist values, prohibiting them from engaging in cooperative organization in the workplace, are also partially correct. These analyses refer, however, only to that segment of white collar workers in a high class position who have chosen the strategy of professionalization--monopoly control over the occupation's education and market.

This study has contributed to the literature on the politics of white collar workers by providing conceptual clarification of their different objective class positions, amplifying on abstract theory by grounding it in empirical study. In addition, it has attempted to transcend generalizations on the white collar workers' subjective dimension by examining the very way in which class position is linked to thought and action. As Katznelson warned, "If social classes are objectively defined locations in the class structure and if people are thus bearers of class relations, they are reduced, in Gordon Marshall's words, to the status of simple executants of strategies imposed on them by the system" (Katznelson, 1986).

I have attempted to avoid such a pitfall and instead have examined the powerful, intervening role of ideology. As Geertz eloquently stated, "It is through the construction of ideologies, schematic images of social order, that man makes himself . . . a political animal" (Geertz, 1973).

NOTE

1.   Trade unions are viewed as significant indicators of class consciousness in this study. As A. R. Luria noted, "Even the lowest level of trade union involvement demands a social practice that challenges, as nothing else, the assumptions of individualism and creates a quite new context for the formulation of concepts and attitudes. . . .   The collectivism inherent in trade union activity is seen as indispensable for the creation of a basic class consciousness that can, in the course of struggle and sometimes with surprising speed, be transformed into a consciousness of a much higher political level" (Fantasia, 1988: 19).

Appendix A

Professional Nurse Survey

The first set of questions I am going to ask have to do with your work.

1. Can you tell me how long you've worked at Mt. Zion/St. John's Hospital?
2. Which unit have you worked on over the past year?
3. Considering ALL the tasks you do on a regular basis, would you describe a typical workday for me, from your entrance to your exit out the hospital door. (I'm interested in EVERYTHING, from taking pulse rates, counseling patients, changing linens, collecting specimens, to making budget decisions.)
4. Do you happen to feel you need any additional education for any of these aspects of your work?   Yes ( ) No ( )
   If yes, what kind of education, and for what purpose?
5. Do you happen to use any special equipment (e.g., an EMG machine or mechanical ventilator) on a regular basis?   Yes ( ) No ( )
   IF NOT, GO ON TO QUESTION 8
   a) Which instrument(s) do you use?
6. Do you happen to think working with special equipment increases, decreases, or does not affect the number of patients you see each day?
7. Do you happen to think working with special equipment affects the quality of patient care you are able to deliver--that is, improve, detract from, or not affect it?   Yes ( ) No ( )
   If improve or detract from, in what way?
8. Do you happen to know whether other health care providers at your hospital perform some of the same tasks as you do (such as technician respiratory therapists, LPNs, or social workers)?   Yes ( ) No ( )
   a)   If yes, what are some of the tasks both YOU and OTHERS perform?
   b)   What are the titles of the others performing them (e.g., social worker)?
   c)   Do you have any say about who else performs these tasks?
                                      Yes ( ) No ( )

If yes, in what way?

9. Did you ever perform any nursing task(s) that you NO LONGER perform because other health care providers now perform such tasks (e.g., in some hospitals, nurses no longer provide anesthesia; doctors do)?

Yes ( ) No ( )

a) If yes, which tasks did you previously perform that are now performed by someone else?

b) What is the title of the other person(s) performing these tasks (e.g., doctor)?

10. What is your current job title (e.g., head nurse)?

11. Which of the following would you say best describes your position in the hospital?
   a) Managerial
   b) Supervisory
   c) Nonmanagerial
   d) Other; please explain

12. If managerial, would that be:
   a) Top manager
   b) Upper manager
   c) Middle manager
   d) Lower manager

13. I'm going to ask you whether you participate in any of the following policy decisions on your job. If you do, would you specify the role you play in each? That is, do you decide jointly with everyone else, make decisions subject to a superior's approval, or make decisions with the final decision up to you?

	Decide with Everyone Else	Make Decision Subject to Approval	Make Final Decision

a) Do you determine the overall size of budget in your department?
   No ( ) ( )   ( )   ( )
b) Do you allocate parts of the budget in your unit?
   No ( ) ( )   ( )   ( )
c) Do you purchase products for your unit?
   No ( ) ( )   ( )   ( )
d) Do you hire or fire employees in your unit?
   No ( ) ( )   ( )   ( )
e) Do you determine the staffing pattern in your unit?
   No ( ) ( )   ( )   ( )

14. Do you supervise anyone on your job?

Yes ( ) No ( )

If yes,

a) Are they other health care workers or support staff such as clerical
    workers?

    Yes ( ) No ( )

b) Can you influence the pay scale or the promotion of those you supervise?

    Yes ( ) No ( )

c) Who would you say has greater influence on promotions and salaries: you
    or someone higher up?

    Yes ( ) No ( )

15. Would you say there are ways you can improve the quality of patient care you
    deliver without consulting a superior?

    Yes ( ) No ( )

    If yes, please describe these.

16. Did you ever happen to participate in an administrative body (within or outside
    your hospital) that shapes nursing standards or policy on education or practice?

    Yes ( ) No ( )

    If yes, which organization was it? Did you participate as a convention delegate,
    a voting member, a board member, or in some other capacity?

17. Now I'd like to ask you some questions about events at Mt. Zion/(St. John's
    Hospital). As you know, there was a decertification attempt of NYSNA for UFT
    in November 1982 (of 1199 for NYSNA).

    Did you happen to agree or disagree with that attempted decertification?

    Agree ( ) Disagree ( )

    Why? That is, what would you say were the greatest advantages of
    (for Mt. Zion Hospital):

        NYSNA over UFT?
        UFT over NYSNA?
    (St. John's Hospital):

        1199 over NYSNA?
        NYSNA over 1199?

18. Many people have strong feelings one way or another about being represented by
    a trade union. Would you say you have such strong feelings?

    Yes ( ) No ( )

    If yes, are they positive or negative?

    Positive ( ) Negative ( )

    What do you see as positive or negative about being represented by a trade
    union?

19. Here are some opinions that others have expressed in connection with trade
    unions. Could you tell me whether you generally agree or disagree with each
    one?

a) Trade unions are corrupt.

    Agree ( ) Disagree ( )

b) Trade unions should be for both blue and white collar workers.

    Agree ( ) Disagree ( )

c)   Trade unions increase the "professionalism" of their members by legally protecting their right to greater responsibility on the job.

                                              Agree ( )   Disagree ( )
d)   Trade unions are too militant in their tactics to represent nurses.

                                              Agree ( )   Disagree ( )
e)   Trade unions and "professionalism" are compatible.

                                              Agree ( )   Disagree ( )

20. Now I'd like to ask you a question on which there is considerable difference of opinion, that is, what constitutes increased professionalism in work? For each of the following activities I mention, which category do you happen to think best describes it for nursing, according to YOUR OWN opinion?
     a)   Having more autonomy over your own work
     b)   Earning a salary comparable to physicians
     c)   Having more supervisory activities over other health care workers
     d)   Having more direct patient care responsibilities
     e)   Having more teaching responsibilities
     f)   Having a baccalaureate degree
     g)   Having more practical experience in combination with any type of RN credential
     h)   Improving the quality of patient care delivery by going on strike if necessary
     i)   If none of the above, how would you define it?

21. Now I'm going to ask you some questions on how you feel about certain aspects of your work, that is, which are important to you?
     a)   How important would you say your SALARY is to you?
          Not important ( ) Somewhat important ( ) Very ( ) Most important ( )
          How would you rate your salary?
          Very good ( )   Good ( )   Fair ( )   Poor ( )
     b)   How important to you is having the ability to make independent decisions about your work without consulting a superior, that is having AUTONOMY?
          Not important ( ) Somewhat important ( ) Very ( ) Most important ( )
          How would you rate the autonomy you have?
          Very good ( )   Good ( )   Fair ( )   Poor ( )
     c)   How important to you is having a PRESTIGIOUS job?
          Not important ( ) Somewhat important ( ) Very ( ) Most important ( )
          How would you rate the prestige of your current job?
          Very good ( )   Good ( )   Fair ( )   Poor ( )
     d)   How important to you is having formal protection from your superiors if you needed it, that is, having set GRIEVANCE PROCEDURES?
          Not important ( ) Somewhat important ( ) Very ( ) Most important ( )
          How would you rate the amount of protection from superiors you have currently?
          Very good ( )   Good ( )   Fair ( )   Poor ( )

e)   How important to you is having a good STAFF-PATIENT ratio on your unit?

Not important ( ) Somewhat important ( ) Very ( ) Most important ( )

How would you rate the current staff-patient ratio on your unit?

Very good ( )   Good ( )   Fair ( )   Poor ( )

f)   How about JOB SECURITY? How important is this to you?

Not important ( ) Somewhat important ( ) Very ( ) Most important ( )

 How would you rate your current job security?

Very good ( )   Good ( )   Fair ( )   Poor ( )

22. Considering the items I just mentioned, such as salary and autonomy, with whom would you say you share such concerns in common? That is, would you say you share concerns about job security, salary, opportunity for advancement, autonomy, protection from superiors, prestige, or staff-patient ratios with:

a)   Hospital technicians

b)   Nursing educators

c)   Nurses' aides

d)   Physicians

e)   LPNs

f)   Nursing administrators

g)   Hospital social workers

If you could change careers tomorrow, would you?

Yes ( ) No ( )

If yes, what would you choose, and why?

Finally, in order to compare what you say with other RNs, the rest of my questions have to do with basic personal information.

23. Are you an RN?

a)   Yes ( )

b)   No ( )

24. Which of the following have you received:

a)   Associate degree   ( )

b)   Diploma   ( )

c)   B.S.N.   ( )

d)   Master's degree   ( )

e)   Ph.D.   ( )

25. What is the highest educational level you completed?

26. If you are married or living with a spouse equivalent,

a)   What is the highest educational level he/she completed?

b)   What is his/her occupation?

27. What is your ethnic group?

a)   Hispanic   ( )

b)   Asian   ( )

c)   White   ( )

     d)   Black   ( )
     e)   Other   ( )

28. What is your sex?
    a)   Male   ( )
    b)   Female   ( )
29. What is your age?
    a)   20-25   ( )
    b)   26-35   ( )
    c)   36-45   ( )
    d)   Above 46   ( )
30. Where is the single place you spent most of your childhood (City and state)?
31. Is your marital status single, married, widowed, separated, divorced, or are you living with a spouse equivalent?
32. What is your yearly salary?
33. What is your total family income?
34. Do you and your family receive income from any other sources, such as:
    a)   Your own family business   ( )
    b)   A government pension   ( )
    c)   Inheritance (over $1000/year)   ( )
    d)   Investments (over $1000/year)   ( )
    e)   Social Security   ( )
    f)   Other   ( )
35. Do you see yourself as belonging to any of the following social classes: the upper class, the middle class, the working class, or some other class?
36. How do you determine your social class?

I want to thank you very much for your time and effort in answering this survey. If you have any comments about the issues covered or the way in which they were covered, please include them.

Appendix B

Survey Coding

CATEGORY OF VARIABLE

1. Class Location
   Economic control   3, 8, 9, 13e, 16
   Political control   13d, 14a-c
   Ideological control   15, 5, 6, 7
   Class location correlated with job title   10, 11, 12
   Income components   32-34
2. Collective Strategy
   Trade unionism   17, 18a-c
   Professional unionism   17
   Professionalization   17, 4
3. Symbol of Professionalism
   Control over conditions of work   19a,d; 20b-g
   Greater respect   19 open ended
   Greater social and economic status   19b,c,f; 20a,d
   Human capital   19 open ended
   Proper behavior   19 open ended
4. Class Identity
   Worker   21a,c,e
   Professional   21b,d,f,g,
   Management   21d,f
   Self-identified class   35-36 open ended
5. Work History
   Years in current position   2
   Years at current workplace   1
   Previous experience   open ended throughout
6. Demographic data   23-31

CODING OF VARIABLES

Category	Variable	Question	Col.	Item	Code
Work history		1	01	Time in hospital	0 0-3 years 1 4-7 years 2 8-over years
Work history		1a	02	Time as nurse	0 0-3 years 1 4-7 years 2 8-over years
Class position		2	03	Unit works in	0 generalized unit 1 specialized unit 2 administration
Class position	Economic control	3	04	Tasks	0 nonspecialized 1 specialized (e.g., ICU)
Class position	Ideological control	5	06	Use specialized equipment	0 yes (low tech.) 1 no (high tech.)
Class position	Ideological control	6	07	Cause speed up?	0 decreases 1 increases 2 no effect on speed
Class position		7	08	omit	
Class position	Economic control	8	09	re-skilling de-skilling	0 no 1 yes 2 w/other types of nurses 3 w/other occupations
			10		

148

CODING OF VARIABLES cont'd

Category	Variable	Question	Col.	Item	Code
Class position	Economic control	9	11	re-skilling	0 no
				de-skilling	1 yes
			12		2 w/other types of nurses
					3 w/other occupations
Class position	Job title	10	13	indicated by job title	0 staff worker
					1 middle management
					2 administration
Class identity		11	14	subjective perception of class position	0 work
					1 management
					2 middle management
Class identity		12	15	subjective perception of class position (if management)	0 low management
					1 middle management
					2 high management
Class position	Political control	13d	16	Control over political level (hire or fire)	0 no control
					1 partial control
					2 full control
Class position	Political control	13e	17	Control over political level (determine staff)	0 no control
					1 partial control
					2 full control
Class position	Political control	14	18	Control over others (supervisory)	0 no control
					1 partial control
					2 full control

CODING OF VARIABLES cont'd

Category	Variable	Question	Col.	Item	Code
Class position	Ideological control	15	19	Control over quality of work	0 no control 1 partial control 2 full control
Class position	Ideological control	16	20	Control over goals and purposes of work	0 no control 1 partial control 2 full control
Collective strategy	Unionization	17	21	Want any type of union	0 no 1 yes
		17	22	If no, why?	0 unions unprof. 1 unions violent
		17	23	If yes, what type?	0 prof. union 1 trade union
Collective strategy	Unionization	17	24	If prof. union, what issues?	0 control over conds. of work 1 control over quality of care (ability to provide good care) 2 status (prestige, money, power) 3 human capital
Collective strategy	Unionization	17	25	If prof. union, what consciousness?	0 "status cons." (reject solidarity w/other workers)

150

CODING OF VARIABLES cont'd

Category	Variable	Question	Col.	Item	Code
					1 "class cons." (seek solidarity w/other workers, needs are in opposition to management) 2 status and class consciousness (see solidarity w/other RNs only, but see staff RNs' needs in opp. to management
Collective strategy	Unionism	18b	26	If trade union, what pos. issues	0 control over work 1 qual. of care 2 status 3 human capital
Class identity	Consciousness	18-2	27	What neg. issues?	0 status 1 class
		18-4	27	What cons.?	0 status 1 class
		18-5	29	What cons.?	0 status 1 class

151

CODING OF VARIBLES cont'd

Category	Variable	Question	Col.	Item	Code
Symbol of the professional	Professionalism	19	30	Its meaning	0 control over work (A,D,E,G,H) 1 status (B,C,F)
			31		0 behavior: "human capital" (improve self-attributes) 1 "proper" behavior (don't strike, etc.)
Demographics		27	46	Ethnicity	0 Hispanic 1 Asian 2 white 3 black
		28	47	Sex	0 male 1 female
		29	48	Age	0 20-25 1 26-35 2 36-45 3 above 46
	Origins	30	49	Where grew up?	0 small town 1 suburbia 2 rural farm 3 urban area 4 country other than U.S.

CODING OF VARIABLES cont'd

Category	Variable	Question	Col.	Item	Code
Origins		31	50	Marital status	0 single 1 married 2 widowed 3 divorced 4 separated 5 living with spouse equivalent
	Salary	32	51	Yearly salary	0 $15,000-19,999 1 $20,000-24,999 2 $25,000-29,999 3 $30,000-34,999 4 $35,000 and above
		33	52	Total family income	0 $15,000-19,999 1 $20,000-24,999 2 $25,000-29,000 3 $30,000-34,999 4 $35,000-39,999 5 $40,000-44,999 6 $45,000-49,999 7 $50,000 and above
Class Position	Objective class position	34	53	Components of income	0 own a family business 1 government assistance 2 family wealth (inheritance)

CODING OF VARIABLES cont'd

Category	Variable	Question	Col.	Item	Code
					3 investments
					4 none
					5 child support, etc.
					6 other job
Class identity		35	54	What class do you see yourself in?	0 working class
					1 middle class
					2 upper class
					3 other

Appendix C

New York State Nurses Association: Questions and Answers about Entry into Practice

At the October 1975 Convention of the New York State Nurses Association, the Voting Body passed a legislative proposal to implement the 1974 Resolution on Entry into Professional Practice through Revision of Article 139, Nursing, Title VIII, Education Law (*The Nurse Practice Act*). This legislative proposal has been placed before each Convention Voting Board since that date and has overwhelmingly passed each time.

The Entry Into Practice Proposal has engendered some questions and misconceptions among nurses and the general public. These questions and answers have been prepared to provide some pertinent facts about the proposal.

1. Q. What is the primary intent of the Entry Into Practice Proposal?
    A. To clarify, standardize and elevate the educational requirements for the legal practice of professional nursing and practical nursing.
2. Q. Specifically, what does this mean?
    A. It means that four years after the bill becomes a law, persons taking the professional nurse licensing examination must have completed a baccalaureate degree program in nursing. Persons taking the associate nurse licensing examination must have completed an associate degree program in nursing.
3. Q. How will the proposal affect individuals currently licensed as registered nurses and practical nurses?
    A. The proposal contains a grandfather mechanism which protects all RNs and LPNs licensed *prior to the date the bill becomes law.*
4. Q. Specifically, what does the grandfather clause provide?
    A. 1) All RNs and LPNs licensed prior to the date the bill becomes law will NOT have to meet the educational requirements specified in the new law.
        2) Those who were licensed as registered professional nurses prior to

that date will retain their *licenses as nurses*.

3) Those who were licensed as LPNs prior to that date will be authorized to use the title *associate nurse*.

(The only way a license can be "taken away" is by the Board of Regents in disciplinary proceedings involving misconduct.)

5. Q.   Is this the first time a grandfather mechanism for nurses will be used in New York State?

   A.   No. It was used in 1903 when the first Nurse Practice Act went into effect (and covered thousands of individuals), and it has been used in every revision thereafter involving qualifications for practice.

6. Q.   It has been said that by "Grandfathering" present RNs and LPNs standards of care will be threatened. Is this true?

   A.   No. Nurses support maintenance of high standards of nursing care and will be assisted in this transition as needed through inservice education.

7. Q.   What has NYSNA done to prepare for implementation?

   A.   In 1977, three task forces were appointed to study the implementation process. Their reports are now final and address these issues:

   1) Identification of the Behavioral Outcomes of the nurse and associate nurse.

   2) Identification of ways to assist the registered nurse in the transition (grandfathering) to the professional nurse.

   3) Identification of ways to assist the licensed practical nurse in the transition (grandfathering) to the associate nurse.

   The three task forces sought and obtained input from nurses across the state. Further, the Council on Legislation has offered its services to speak with District Nurse's Associations, Councils of Nursing Practitioners, students in schools of nursing and others.

8. Q.   What impact will the entry into practice bill have on career mobility?

   A.   It will promote career mobility. The present chaotic system of nursing education does not maximize potential for long range career planning and educational mobility. It has resulted in confusion and frustration among many graduates of the various kinds of nursing programs. For years those RNs and LPNs who wanted to change their career patterns have either been rejected, or have been forced to spend inordinate time, energy and money in reaching their career goals.

   This legislation will provide for two careers in nursing, each with its own distinct and standardized educational requirement. With this new system of basic nursing education, we can minimize these present barriers to true career mobility:

   1) Inappropriate and misleading counselling of students seeking admission into schools of nursing;

   2) Frustration of graduates of schools of nursing seeking further

preparation;

3) Difficulty in transferring credits between nursing education programs and between nursing and other education programs.

9. Q.   Why are changes needed in the educational qualifications for the practice of nursing?

   A.   1) The ongoing major advances in health science and technology demand ongoing changes in the educational preparation of health practitioners in order to meet society's health needs.

        2) The present system of nursing education is chaotic and costly--three different kinds of programs prepare the registered nurse and a variety of programs prepare the practical nurse.

        3) Nursing is the only major health occupation which does not require a minimum of a baccalaureate degree for entry into professional practice.

10. Q. What impact will the entry into practice requirements have on interstate mobility?

    A. If New York State or any other state passes the Entry Into Practice Law (many other states have endorsed similar resolutions and are moving toward legislation), *in keeping with present laws*, any RN or LPN transferring from one state to another will need to meet the licensure requirements in effect in the new state.   Authority for licensing professions rests with state governments. Because of diversity among the states, each state must develop legislation to meet its particular social, economic and educational needs.

        Although all Nurse Practice Acts in the fifty states were not established at the same time in history, nor are they exactly the same today, the nursing profession has developed mechanisms to foster interstate mobility.

        Given the current national interest in clarifying the existing system of nursing education and licensure, it is reasonable to expect that the nursing profession will again foster interstate mobility.

11. Q. Concern has been raised about the costs involved in requiring baccalaureate degrees for professional nurses and associate degrees for practical nurses.

    A. These facts should be considered in the issue of costs:

        1) Two year (community college) nursing programs would be eligible for federal vocational education funds that presently support practical nursing education.

        2) If nursing education is brought into the mainstream of higher education, it will be sharing in the abundant resources of the state's public and independent academic institutions rather than maintaining separate, costly educational facilities (library resources, teaching equipment, classroom space, and support

personnel).

3) The cost of nursing education should be borne by educational institutions, be they public or independent, and not by service institutions which rely on insurance reimbursement monies to subsidize the cost of educating students, making the cost of health insurance higher than necessary.

12. Q.   How will this legislation affect the current shortage of nurses? Won't it become worse?

A.   Numerous studies have found the "nursing shortage" to be a result of increased utilization of nurses, dissatisfaction on the part of nurses with working conditions, lack of nursing input in health care decision making, lack of respect for nursing on the part of professional colleagues, and poor salaries. School of Nursing enrollment trends show that fewer individuals are selecting nursing as a career. Standardizing and elevating nursing education is the only way to reverse these trends. Nursing must become a profession equal in status to the other health professions in image, input and rewards for nursing to be an attractive career choice for today's young women and men.

13. Q.   Hasn't the issue of entry into nursing practice been around for a long time?

A.   Indeed.

The history of nursing, from Nightingale to the present, is replete with efforts by nurses to truly "professionalize" the occupation of nursing. During the past seventy-five years, innumerable studies, investigations, reports and recommendations have been produced relative to a desirable system of nursing education.

In 1965, the American Nurses' Association issued its position paper declaring that minimum preparation for beginning professional nursing practice should be the baccalaureate degree in nursing and that minimum preparation for beginning technical nursing practice should be the associate degree in nursing. NYSNA, following ANA's leadership, issued *A Blueprint for the Education of Nurses in New York State* in 1967 stating a plan for the orderly transition of nursing education in New York State into the mainstream of higher education.

Clearly, it is time for immediate action to get on with the task at hand--namely, the professionalization of nursing.

References

Aiken, Linda. 1983. "Challenges of Hospital Nursing." In Linda Aiken (ed.), *Nursing in the 80's: Crises, Opportunities and Challenges.* Philadelphia: Lippincott.

Alford, Robert. 1975. *Health Care Politics: Ideological and Interest Group Barriers to Reform.* Chicago: University of Chicago Press.

American Hospital Association. 1989. *Guide to the Health Care Field.* Chicago: American Hospital Association.

American Journal of Nursing. 1984. "Entry Level Legislation May Be Reachable," 6:832.

_____. 1983. "Staff Cutbacks Are Hurting Nursing Services as Pressures Mount to Hold Down Hospital Spending" (June).

American Nurses Association. 1983. "Testimony of ANA on the Reauthorization of the Federal Trade Commission." U.S. Senate, Commission on Commerce, Science and Transportation, March 17.

_____. 1979. "A Case for Baccalaureate Preparation for Nursing." Kansas City, Mo.: ANA.

_____. 1965. "Educational Preparation for Nurses: A Position Paper." Kansas City, Mo.: ANA.

_____. 1965. *Educational Preparation for Nurse Practitioners and Assistants to Nurses: A Position Paper.* New York: AMNA.

Annual Report. 1970; 1981; 1983; 1986; 1989. New York: Mt. Zion Hospital (a pseudonym).

Annual Report. 1976. "The First 125 Years." New York: Mt. Zion Hospital (a pseudonym).

Appelbaum, Eileen, and Cherlyn Granrose. 1986. "Hospital Employment under Revised Medicare Payment Schedules," *Monthly Labor Review* (August).

Aronowitz, Stanley. 1983. *Working Class Hero: A New Strategy for Labor.* New York: Pilgrim Press.

Backup, Molly, and John Molinaro. 1984. "New Health Professionals: Changing the Hierarchy." In Victor Sidel and Ruth Sidel (eds.), *Reforming Medicine.* New York: Pantheon.

Bell, Daniel. 1973. *The Coming of Post-Industrial Society: A Venture in Social*

Forecasting. New York: Basic Books.

Bellaby, Paul, and Patrick Oribabor. 1977. "Growth of Trade Union Consciousness among General Hospital Nurses Viewed As a Response to Proletarianization." *Sociological Review* 25 (4).

Bellah, Robert, Richard Madsen, William Sullivan, Ann Swidler, and Steven Tipton. 1985. *Habits of the Heart: Individualism and Commitment in American Life.* Berkeley: University of California Press.

Benson, Susan Porter. 1984. "Women in Retail Saleswork: The Continuing Dilemma of Service." In Karen Sacks and Dorothy Remey (eds.), *My Troubles Are Going to Have Trouble with Me.* New Brunswick, N.J.: Rutgers University Press.

_____. 1978. "The Clerking Sisterhood: Rationalization and the Work Culture of Saleswomen." *Radical America* 12 (2).

Berg, Barbara. 1978. *The Remembered Gate: Origins of American Feminism: The Woman and the City, 1800-1860.* New York: Oxford University Press.

Bluestone, Barry, and Bennett Harrison. 1988. *The Great Un-Turn.* New York: Basic Books.

_____. 1982. *Deindustrialization.* New York: Basic Books.

Bowles, Samuel, and Herbert Gintis. 1976. *Schooling in Capitalist America: Educational Reform and the Contradictions of Economic Life.* New York: Basic Books.

Braverman, Harry. 1974. *Labor and Monopoly Capital: The Degradation of Work in the Twentieth Century.* New York: Monthly Review Press.

Brint, Steven. 1986. *Professional Workers and Unionization: A Data Handbook.* Washington, D.C.: Department for Professional Employees, AFL-CIO.

Brint, Steven, and J. Karabel. 1989. *The Diverted Dream: Community Colleges and the Promise of Educational Opportunities in America, 1900-1985.* New York: Oxford University Press.

Brown, Carol. 1973. "The Division of Laborers: Allied Health Professionals." *International Journal of Health Services* 3 (3).

Brown, Esther Lucille. 1948. *Nursing for the Future.* Troy, N.Y.: Russell Sage Foundation.

Brown, Richard. 1979. *Rockefeller Medicine Men.* Berkeley: University of California.

Brown, Susan, 1980. "The Professionalization and Unionization of Nurses." Unpublished paper, University of South Carolina, Columbia.

Brumberg, Joan, and Nancy Tomes. 1982. "Women in the Professions." *Reviews of American History* (Fall-Summer).

Burawoy, Michael. 1979. *Manufacturing Consent: Changes in the Labor Process under Capitalism.* Chicago: University of Chicago Press.

_____. 1978. "Braverman and Beyond." *Politics and Society* 8 (3).

Campbell, Marie. 1987a. "Management as 'Ruling': A Class Phenomenon in Nursing." Unpublished manuscript.

_____. 1987b. "Productivity in Canadian Nursing: Administering Cuts." In David Coburn (ed.), *Health and Canadian Society: Sociological Perspectives.* Markham, Ontario: Fitzheury and Whiteside.

_____. 1987c. "Accounting for Care: A Framework for Analyzing Change in Canadian Nursing." In Rosemary White (ed.), *Political Issues in Nursing*, vol. 3. New York: Wiley.

Cannings, Kathleen, and William Lazonick. 1975. "The Development of the Nursing

Laborforce in the U.S.: A Basic Analysis." *International Journal of Health Services* 5 (2).

Clark, Sondra. 1985. Personal communication, former head of RN Division, Local 1199.

____. 1979. "Nurses to ANA Proposal: No Way!" *1199 News* (March):23.

Cohen, Abner. 1979. "Political Symbolism." *Annual Review of Anthropology:*87-113.

Collins, Randall. 1979. *The Credential Society: An Historical Sociology of Education and Stratification.* New York: Academic Press.

Cooper, Joseph. 1987. "White Collar Salaries Vary Widely in the Service Industries." *Monthly Labor Review* (November) 110:21-23.

Corey, Lewis. 1935. *The Crisis of the Middle Class.* New York: Covici, Friede.

Davies, Margery. 1982. *Woman's Place Is at the Typewriter: Office Work and Office Workers, 1870-1930.* Philadelphia: Temple University Press.

Denton, David Rehmi. 1976. "The Union Movement in American Hospitals." Ph.D. thesis, Boston University.

Derber, Charles. 1983. "Managing Professionals: Ideological Proletarianization and Post Industrial Labor." *Theory and Society* (May).

____ (ed.). 1982. *Professionals as Workers: Mental Labor in Advanced Capitalism.* Boston: G. K. Hall.

Dolan, Andrew. 1979a. "Nursing's Quest for Identity." *Health/PAC Bulletin,* 81, 82.

____. 1979b. "The New York State Nurses Association 1985 Proposal: Who Needs It?" *Journal of Health Politics and Law* 2 (4).

Donaldson, Bessie. 1933. *The Long Island College Hospital and Training School for Nurses, 1858-1933.* Brooklyn, N.Y.: Willis McDonald & Co.

Eckholm, Erik (ed.). 1993. *Solving America's Health Care Crisis.* New York: Random House.

Edwards, Richard. 1979. *Contested Terrain: The Transformation of the Workplace in the Twentieth Century.* New York: Basic Books.

Edwards, Richard, Michael Reich, and David Gordon. 1975. *Labor Market Segmentation.* Lexington, Mass.: D. C. Health.

Ehrenreich, Barbara, and John Ehrenreich. 1979. "The Professional Managerial Class." In Pat Walker (ed.), *Between Labor and Capital.* Boston: South End Press.

____. 1976. "Work and Consciousness." *Monthly Review* (July-August) 28 (3).

____. 1971. *The American Health Empire: Power, Profits and Politics. A Report from the Health Policy Advisory Center.* New York: Vintage Books.

Epstein, Barbara. 1982. "Industrialization and Feminization: A Case Study of 19th Century New England." In Rachel Kahn-Hut et al. (eds.), *Women and Work.* New York: Oxford University Press.

Etzioni, Amitai. 1969. *The Semi-Professions and Their Organization.* New York: Free Press.

Fantasia, Rick. 1988. *Cultures of Solidarity: Consciousness, Action and Contemporary American Workers.* Berkeley: University of California Press.

Feldberg, Roslyn, and Evelyn Nakano Glen. 1981. "Male and Female: Job Versus Gender Models in the Sociology of Work." In Rachel Kahn-Hut et al. (eds.), Women and Work. New York: Oxford University Press.

Ferree, Myra Mary. 1989. "Family and Job for Working Class Women: Gender and Class Systems See from Below." In Naomi Gerstel and Harriet Gross (eds.), *Family and Work*. Philadelphia: Temple University Press.

Fink, Leon. 1986. "Bread and Roses, Crusts and Thorns: The Troubled Story of 1199." *Dissent* (Spring).

Fink, Leon, and Brian Greenberg. 1989. *Upheaval in the Quiet Zone: A History of Hospital Workers' Union Local 1199*. Urbana: University of Illinois.

Freeman, Richard, and Leonard, Jonathan. 1987. "Union Maids: Unions and the Female Workforces." In Clair Brown and Joseph Pechmen (eds.), *Gender in the Workplace*. Washington, D.C.: Brookings Institute.

Friedson, Eliot. 1975. *Doctoring Together*. New York: Elsevier.

_____. 1973a. "Professionalization and the Organization of Middle Class Labor in Post-Industrial Society." In Paul Halmos (ed.), *Professionalization and Social Change: The Sociology Review*, no. 20, Keele, England: University of Keele.

_____. 1973b. "Professions and the Occupational Principle." In E. Friedson (Ed.), *The Professions and Their Prospects*. Beverly Hills, Calf.: Sage Publishers.

_____. 1970. *The Profession of Medicine: A Study of the Sociology of Applied Knowledge*. New York: Dodd, Mead.

Gans, Herb. 1988. *Middle American Individualism: The Future of Liberal Democracy*. New York: Free Press.

Geertz, Clifford. 1973. "Ideology as a Cultural System." In *The Interpretation of Cultures*. New York: Basic Books.

_____. 1964. "Ideology as a Belief System." In David Apter (ed.), *Ideology and Discontent*. New York: Free Press.

Gilbert, Susan. 1990. "Is America Abandoning Sick Patients?" *New York Times, The Good Health Magazine*, April 29, 1990, 23, 30, 33.

Gintis, Herb. 1970. "The New Working Class and Revolutionary Youth," *Socialist Review*1 (3):13-43.

Goldmark, Josephine. 1928. *Nursing and Nursing Education in the United States: Report on the Committee for the Study of Nursing Education*. New York: Macmillan.

Gordon, David M., Richard Edwards, and Michael Reich. 1982. *Segmented Work, Divided Workers: The Historical Transformation of Labor in the U.S.* Cambridge: Cambridge University Press.

Gorz, Andre. 1980. *Farewell to the Working Class*. Boston: South End Press.

_____. 1976. "Technology, Technicians and Class Struggle." In André Gorz (ed.), *The Division of Labor*. Atlantic Highlands, N.J.: Humanities Press.

_____. 1972. "Technical Intelligence and the Capitalist Division of Labor." *Telos* 12 (Summer).

_____. 1967. *Strategy for Labor*. Boston: Beacon Press.

Gouldner, Alvin. 1979. *The Future of Intellectuals and the Rise of the New Class*. London: Macmillan.

Gouldner, F. H., and R. Ritti. 1967. "Professionalism as Career Immobility." *American Journal of Sociology*, 489-502.

Gramsci, Antonio. 1971. *Prison Notebooks*. New York: International Publishers.

Gutman, Herb. 1976. *Work, Culture and Society in Industrializing America: Essays in American Working Class and Social History*. New York: Knopf.

Halle, David. 1984. *America's Working Man: Work, Home and Politics among Blue Collar Property Owners*. Chicago: University of Chicago Press.

Halle, David, and Peter Romo. 1991. "The Blue Collar Working Class: Continuity and

Change." In Alan Wolfe (ed.), *America at Century's End*. Berkeley: University of California Press.

Hareven, Tamara. 1982. *Family Time and Industrial Time*. New York: Cambridge University Press.

Hareven, Tamara, and Maris Vinovski. 1975. "Marital Fertility, Ethnicity and Occupation in Urban Families: An Analysis of South Boston and the South End in 1880." *Journal of Social History* 3 (Spring).

Himmelstein, David, and Steffi Woolhandler. 1984. "Medicine as Industry: The Health-Care Sector in the United States." *Monthly Review* 35 (April).

Hirsch, J., and B. Dougherty. 1952. *The First 100 Years: The Mount Sinai Hospital of New York, 1852-1952*. New York: Random House.

Hofstadter, Richard. 1955. *The Age of Reform: From Bryan to FDR*. New York: Knopf.

Hughes, E. C. 1958. *Men and Their Work*. New York: Free Press.

Immergut, Ellen M. 1982. "Doctors and the State." Unpublished manuscript. Department of Sociology, Harvard University.

Institute of Medicine. 1983. *Nursing and Nursing Education: Public Policies and Private Actions*. Washington, D.C.: National Academy Press.

James, Janet. 1979. "Isabel Hampton and the Professionalization of Nursing in the 1890s." In Charles Rosenberg and Morris Vogel (eds.), *The Therapeutic Revolution*. Philadelphia: University of Pennsylvania Press.

Johnson, T. J. 1977. "The Professions in the Class Structure." In R. Scase (ed.), *Industrial Society: Class Cleavage and Control*. London: Allen and Unwin.

Karabel, Jerome. 1972. "Community Colleges and Social Stratification." *Harvard Education Review* 42 (4) (November).

Katznelson, Ira. 1986. "Working Class Formation: Constructing Cases and Comparisons." In Ira Katznelson and Aristotle Zolberg, *Working Class Formation: Nineteenth Century Patterns in Western Europe and the United States*. Princeton, N.J.: Princeton University Press.

Kerr, Peter. 1993. "Reshaping the Medical Marketplace." *New York Times Magazine*, November 14, 1993, 11.

Kessler-Harris, Alice. 1982. *Out to Work: A History of Wage Earning Women in the United States*. New York: Oxford University Press.

Klein, Joe. 1985. "Labor Pains: Turmoil Grips and Old Left Union." *New York Magazine*, March 25.

Kotelchuck, David. 1976. *Prognosis Negative: Crisis in the Health Care System*. New York: Vintage Books.

Kuttner, Bob. 1984. "Jobs." *Dissent* (Winter).

Lagemann, Ellen (ed.). 1983. *Nursing History: New Perspectives, New Possibilities*. New York: Teachers College Press.

Lamphere, Louise. 1986. "From Working Daughters to Working Mothers: Production and Reproduction in an Industrial Community." *American Ethnologist* 31 (1) (February).

_____. 1985. "Bringing the Family to Work: Women's Culture on the Shop Floor." *Feminist Studies* 11 (3) (Fall).

Larson, Magali S. 1980. "Proletarianization and Educated Labor." *Theory and Society* 9.

_____. 1979. "Professionalism: Rise and Fall." *International Journal of Health*

Services 9 (4).

____. 1977. *The Rise of Professionalism: A Sociological Analysis.* Berkeley: University of California Press.

Lederer, Emil. 1967. *State of the Masses: The Threat of the Classless Society.* New York: Fertig.

Lee, Anthony. 1982. "What Computers Can Do for You and What They're Already Doing for the Lucky Few." *RN Magazine* (September).

____. 1979. "Seven Out of Ten Nurses Oppose the Professional/Technical Split." *RN Magazine* (January).

Levy, Margaret. 1978. "Functional Redundancy and the Process of Professionalization: The Case of the RN's in the United States." Unpublished. Seattle, Wash.: University of Washington.

Lipow, Arthur. 1982. *Authoritarian Socialism in America: Edward Bellamy and the Nationalist Movement.* Berkeley: University of California Press.

Lockhart, Carol Ann, and William Werther. 1980. *Labor Relations in Nursing.* Wakefield, Mass.: Nursing Resources.

Lubove, Roy. 1965. *The Professional Altruist: The Emergence of Social Work as a Career, 1880-1930.* Cambridge: Harvard University Press.

Mallet, Serge. 1975. *Essays on the New Working Class.* St. Louis: Telos Press.

Marmor, Theodore. 1993. "Coalition or Collision? Medicare and Health Reform." *American Prospect* (Winter).

Melosh, Barbara. 1986. "Nursing and Reaganomics: Cost Containment in the United States." In R. White (ed.), *Political Issues in Nursing: Past, Present, and Future,* vol. 2. New York: Wiley.

____. 1982. *The Physician's Hand: Work Culture and Conflict in American Nursing.* Philadelphia: Temple University Press.

Milkman, Ruth. 1993. "Union Responses to Workforce Feminization in the U.S." In Jane Jenson and Mahon Rianne (eds.), *The Challenge of Restructuring.* Temple University Press.

Miller, Richard, Brian Becker, and Edward Krinksy. 1979. *The Impact of Collective Bargaining on Hospitals.* New York: Praeger Press.

Mills, C. Wright. 1951. *White Collar: The American Middle Classes.* New York: Oxford University Press.

Montgomery, David. 1979. *Workers' Control in America.* Cambridge: Cambridge University Press.

Monthly Labor Review. 1987. "Occupational Pay Structure in Nursing and Personal Care Facilities." 110 (41-42) (July).

Morone, James. 1992. "Hidden Complications: Why Health Care Competition Needs Regulation." *American Prospect* (Summer).

Moses, E., and E. Levine. 1983. "RNs Today: A Statistical Profile." In Linda Aiken (ed.), *Nursing in the 80's: Crises, Opportunities and Challenges.* Philadelphia: Lippincott.

Mottus, Jane E. 1980. *New York Nightingales: The Emergence of the Nursing Profession at Bellevue and New York Hospital, 1850-1920.* Ann Arbor: University Microfilms International.

Newman, Katherine. 1993. *Declining Fortunes: The Withering of the American Dream.* New York: Basic Books.

____. 1988. *Falling from Grace: The Experience of Downward Mobility in the*

American Middle Class. New York: Free Press.

———. 1987. "PATCO Lives! Stigma, Heroism and Symbolic Transformations." *Cultural Anthropology* 2 (3).

———. 1986. "Symbolic Dialects and Generations of Women: Variation in the Meaning of Post-Divorce Downward Mobility." *American Ethnologist* 13:230-252.

New York State Education Department. 1983a. "Higher Education Law of New York State 1983 Article 139." In *Candidate Handbook-Nursing*. September. Albany: Division of Professional Licensing Services.

———. 1983b. "Nurse Practice Act and Education Law, Rules and Regulations Pertaining to Nursing in New York State." In *Candidate Handbook-Nursing*. Albany: Division of Professional Licensing Services.

New York State Nurses Association. 1983. "Questions and Answers about Entry into Practice."

———. 1976. Memo to Mt. Zion VP personnel from Deputy Director of NYSNA, December 8.

New York Times. 1988. "AMA Backs New Category of Hospital Worker." Health Pages, June 30.

Noble, David. 1979. "Social Choice in Machine Design: The Case of Automatically Controlled Tools." In A. Zimbalist (ed.), *Case Studies on the Labor Process*. New York: Monthly Review Press.

———. 1977. *America by Design: Science Technology and the Rise of Corporate Capitalism*. New York: Knopf.

O'Connor, James. 1973. *The Fiscal Crisis of the State*. New York: St. Martin's Press.

Oppenheimer, Martin. 1985. *White Collar Politics*. New York: Monthly Review Press.

———. 1975. "The Unionization of the Professional." *Social Policy* (January-February).

———. 1973. "Proletarianization of the Professional." In Paul Halmos (ed.), *Professionalization and Social Change*. Sociological Review Monograph 20. Keele, England: University of Keele.

Phillips, Kevin. 1993. *Boiling Point*. New York: Random House.

Poulantzas, Nicos. 1975. *Classes in Contemporary Capitalism*. London: NLB.

———. 1973. "On Social Classes." *New Left Review,* no. 78 (March-April).

Reich, Robert. 1992. *The Work of Nations*. New York: Vintage Press.

Reverby, Susan. 1987. *Ordered to Care: The Dilemma of American Nursing, 1850-1945*. New York: Cambridge University Press.

———. 1982. "The Nursing Disorder: A Critical History of the Hospital-Nursing Relationship, 1860-1945." Ph.D. thesis. Boston University.

Reverby, Susan, and David Rosner. 1979. *Health Care in America: Essays in Social History*. Philadelphia: Temple University Press.

Rosner, David. 1986. *A Once Charitable Enterprise: Hospitals and Health Care in Brooklyn and New York, 1885-1915*. New York: Cambridge University Press.

Ryan, Mary. 1984. *Cradle of the Middle Class: The Family in Oneida County, New York, 1790-1865*. New York: Cambridge University Press.

Sacks, Karen. 1988. *Caring by the Hour: Women, Work and Organizing at Duke Medical Center*. Urbana: University of Illinois Press.

———. 1984. *My Troubles Are Going to Have Trouble with Me: Everyday Trials and Triumphs of Women Workers*. New Brunswick, N.J.: Rutgers University Press.

Schwartz-Cowan, Ruth. 1983. *More Work for Mother*. New York: Basic Books.

Shapiro-Perl, Nina. 1984. "Resistance Strategies: The Routine Struggle for Bread and

Roses." In K. Sacks (ed.), *My Troubles Are Going to Have Trouble with Me: Everyday Trials and Triumphs of Women Workers*. New Brunswick, N.J.: Rutgers University Press.

Starr, Paul. 1993. "Healthy Compromise: Universal Coverage and Managed Competition under a Cap." *American Prospect* (Winter).

_____. 1982. *The Social Transformation of American Medicine*. New York: Basic Books.

State University of New York Downstate Medical Center. 1960. *Medical Education in Brooklyn, The First Hundred Years, 1860-1960*. Brooklyn, N.Y.: SUNY Downstate Medical Center.

Steinberg, Stephen. 1981. *The Ethnic Myth: Race, Ethnicity, and Class in America*. New York: Atheneum.

Stodder, Jim. 1973. "Old and New Working Class." *Socialist Revolution* 3 (5): 99-100.

Stone, Katherine. 1975. "The Origins of Job Structures in the Steel Industry." In R. Edwards, M. Reich, and D. Gordon (eds.), *Labor Market Segmentation*. Lexington, Mass: D. C. Heath.

Stroeber, Myra. 1984. "Toward a Gender Theory of Occupational Sex Segregation: The Case of Public School Teaching." In Barbara Reskin (ed.), *Sex Segregation in the Workplace*. Washington, D.C.: National Academy Press.

Stroeber, Myra, and Carolyn L. Arnold. 1987. "The Dynamics of Occupational Segregation among Bank Tellers." In C. Brown and J. Peckman (eds.), *Gender in the Workplace*. Washington, D.C.: Brookings Institute.

Survey Research Center. 1977. "Effectiveness in Work Roles: Employee Responses to Work Environment." Ann Arbor, Mich.: Institute for Sociological Research: University of Michigan.

Sweeney, Joan. 1980. "Associate Degree Educator Supports Entry into Practice Resolution." *Nurse Educator* (September-October).

Taylor, Frederick. 1947. *Scientific Management*. New York: Harper.

Tomes, Nancy. 1978. "Little World of Our Own: The Pennsylvania Hospital Training School for Nurses, 1895-1907." *Journal of the History of Medicine and Allied Sciences* 33 (October).

Touraine, Alain. 1971. *The May Movement-Revolt and Reform: May 1968-The Student Rebellion and Workers' Strikes--The Birth of a Social Movement*. New York: Random House.

United States Bureau of Labor Statistics. 1993a. *Professional Specialty Occupations*. Washington, D.C.: Government Printing Office.

_____. 1993b. Bulletin 2400, May 1992-1993. Washington, D.C.: U. S. Government Printing Office.

_____. 1981. *Industry Wage Survey: Hospitals*. Washington, D.C.: U. S. Government Printing Office.

_____. 1963. *Industry Wage Survey*. Washington, D.C.: U. S. Government Printing Office.

United States Department of Commerce, Bureau of the Census. 1976. *Historical Statistics of United States: Colonial Times to 1970*. Washington, D.C.: U. S. Government Printing Office.

_____. 1985. *Statistical Abstract of United States, 1970 and 1980*. Washington, D.C.: U. S. Government Printing Office.

Unity and Progress News. 1984. "RNs Angry--Decerts Wrong Way to Go," (October).

Vanneman, Reeve, and Lynn Weber Cannon. 1987. *The American Perception of Class.* Philadelphia: Temple University Press.

Vesey, Lawrence. 1965. *Emergence of the American University.* Chicago: University of Chicago Press.

Vogel, Morris. 1980. *The Invention of the Modern Hospital, Boston, 1870-1930.* Chicago: University of Chicago Press.

Wagner, David. 1980. "The Proletarianization of Nursing in the United States, 1932-1946." *International Journal of Health Services,* no. 10: 271-90.

White, David. 1984. "Turnergate" audiotape. David White interviewed by Dennis Rivera on Doris Turner.

Wiebe, Robert. 1967. *The Search for Order, 1877-1920.* New York: Hill and Wang.

Wilensky, H. 1964. "The Professionalization of Everyone?" *American Journal of Sociology* (September).

Wilentz, Sean. 1983. "Artisan Republican Festivals and the Rise of Class Conflict in New York City, 1788-1837." In Michael Frisch and Daniel Walkowitz (eds.), *Working Class America.* Urbana: University of Illinois Press.

Wilson, James. 1979. "Isabel Hampton and the Professionalization of Nursing in the 1890's." In M. Vogel and C. Rosenberg (eds.), *The Therapeutic Revolution.* Philadelphia: University of Pennsylvania Press.

Winfield, James MacFarlane. 1915. "The Long Island College Hospital." *New York Medical Journal,* February 13.

Wright, E. O. 1989. *The Debate on Classes.* London: Verso.

____. 1982. "The American Class Structure." *American Sociology Review* 47 (December): 709-726.

____. 1980. "Class and Occupation." *Theory and Society* 9:177-214.

____. 1976. "Class Boundaries in Advanced Capitalist Societies." *New Left Review,* no. 98 (July-August).

Zussman, Robert. 1985. *Mechanics of the Middle Class: Work and Politics among American Engineers.* Berkeley: University of California Press.

Index

American Hospital Association, 19
American Journal of Nursing, 58, 64, 82
American Medical Assn. (AMA), 13, 14, 19, 80, 126
American Nurses Association (ANA), 7, 41, 44, 47, 123
Annual Report, 15, 16, 21
Arnold, Carolyn L., 31
Aronowitz, Stanley, 4

Backup, Molly, 19
Bell, Daniel, 3, 4, 52, 134, 135, 138
Bellaby, Paul, 4
Bellah, Robert, 121, 137
Benson, Susan Porter, 5, 136
Berg, Barbara, 37
blue collar workers, 2-3, 5, 40, 51, 64, 87, 90, 92-93, 105-106, 109, 113, 115, 117, 119, 124, 127, 135, 138
Bluestone, Barry, 2
Bowles, Samuel, 32
Braverman, Harry, 2, 3, 5, 31, 51
Brint, Steven, 32, 47, 59, 73, 79, 99
Brown, Carol, 6
Brown, Esther, 45
Brown, Richard, 13, 14, 16
Burawoy, Michael, 5, 89, 136
Bureau of the Census, 2

Campbell, Marie, 83, 84, 85

Cannon, Lynn Weber, 3
capital individualism, 9, 25, 36, 88, 90-91, 95, 105, 119, 123-125, 127, 129, 136
Civil War, 15, 18, 37, 39, 40
Clark, Sondra, 23, 24, 46, 99
class
    middle class, 3-4, 33-34, 39-41, 52, 74, 121
    new middle class, 3, 40
    new petite bourgeoisie, 3
    new working class, 3, 134
    professionalization, 4, 51
    professional-managerial, 4
    proletarianization, 4
    working class, 3, 10, 32, 35, 37-38, 51-53, 73, 79, 81, 86, 104, 114, 117, 126, 134
class identity, vii, 4-5, 8, 10, 12, 25, 51-53, 87, 89, 93, 106-107, 113, 135-136
    conflicted, 118-119
    consciousness, 4, 10, 52
    with individualized forms of social mobility, 4
    with organized labor, 2, 4, 25
    of professionals, 5
    as working class, 93
class position, 88. *See also* low class position; medium class position; high class position

About the Author

JACQUELINE GOODMAN-DRAPER is an Assistant Professor in the Department of Sociology at State University of New York, Potsdam College. She received a National Science Foundation Award to conduct research for this book and a Nuala McGann Drescher SUNY Award to write it during research leave. She has received numerous other research grants and published several articles.

ISBN 0-86569-248-3

EAN

HARDCOVER BAR CODE

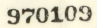